Dosage Dilemmas Deciphered

A Problem-Solving Approach to Pharmaceutical Calculations and Clinical Applications

Gemma Bellweather

Contents

1 Fundamentals of Dosage Calculations

Accurate dosage calculations are the bedrock of safe and effective medication administration. This chapter lays the groundwork for mastering these essential calculations, beginning with a discussion of fundamental units and their conversions. We'll then delve into two primary methods for calculating dosages: ratio and proportion, and dimensional analysis. These tools will empower you to confidently and accurately determine appropriate drug doses across a wide range of clinical scenarios.

The metric system, with its logical and interconnected units, is the cornerstone of pharmaceutical calculations. Familiarity with basic units of weight (grams, milligrams, micrograms, kilograms), volume (liters, milliliters), and length (meters, centimeters, millimeters) is paramount. Equally important is the ability to convert seamlessly between these units. Remember, one gram equals 1000 milligrams, one milligram equals 1000 micrograms, and so on. These conversions are not mere mathematical exercises; they are critical for ensuring that patients receive the correct amount of medication. Imagine the consequences of misinterpreting a dose written in milligrams as micrograms – the difference could be a thousandfold!

Beyond the metric system, you may encounter other units like pounds, ounces, and teaspoons, particularly in home healthcare settings. Converting between these systems requires careful attention. For instance, knowing that one kilogram is approximately equivalent to 2.2 pounds can be crucial when calculating dosages based on a patient's weight. Likewise, understanding that one teaspoon holds approximately 5 milliliters allows for accurate measurement of liquid medications. These seemingly simple conversions are essential building blocks for accurate and safe medication administration.

Once you're comfortable with unit conversions, we move on to ratio and proportion. This method involves setting up two ratios and solving for the unknown quantity. One ratio represents the known drug concentration (e.g., milligrams per milliliter), while the other represents the desired dose and the unknown volume needed to achieve that dose. Cross-multiplication and division are then used to solve for the unknown. This method, while straightforward, requires meticulous attention to units. Ensure that the units in both ratios align to avoid errors. For example, if one ratio uses milligrams, the other must also use milligrams, not micrograms or grams.

Dimensional analysis, also known as the factor-label method, offers a more systematic approach to dosage calculations. This method utilizes conversion factors to cancel out unwanted units and arrive at the desired unit. Each conversion factor represents an equivalent relationship between two units. For example, the conversion factor 1000 mg/1 g can be used to convert grams to milligrams, or its reciprocal, 1 g/1000 mg, to convert milligrams to grams. The beauty of dimensional analysis lies in its ability to handle complex calculations involving multiple conversions. By carefully arranging conversion factors, ensuring that units cancel out appropriately, you can systematically arrive at the correct answer. This method minimizes the risk of errors and provides a clear, auditable trail of your calculations.

Consider the scenario of a physician ordering 250 mg of a medication available as a 125 mg/5 mL solution. Using ratio and proportion, we set up the equation: 125 mg/5 mL = 250 mg/x mL. Cross-multiplying and solving for x reveals that 10 mL of the solution is needed to deliver the prescribed dose. Using dimensional analysis, we can achieve the same result by setting up the calculation as follows: 250 mg * (5 mL/125 mg) = 10 mL. Notice how the milligrams cancel out, leaving us with the desired unit of milliliters.

While both ratio and proportion and dimensional analysis can be used effectively, dimensional analysis is often preferred for complex calculations involving multiple conversions. Its systematic approach and built-in error checking through unit cancellation make it a powerful tool for ensuring accurate dosage calculations. Mastering these fundamental concepts will not only improve your accuracy but also boost your confidence in handling a wide range of dosage calculations. This strong foundation will serve you well as you progress to more advanced concepts and clinical applications later in this book. With consistent practice and attention to detail, you'll be well on your way to becoming proficient in the crucial skill of dosage calculation.

1.1 Units and Conversions

The foundation of accurate drug dosage calculations lies in a thorough understanding of units and their conversions. In the realm of healthcare, precision is paramount, and even seemingly small discrepancies in measurements can have significant consequences. This chapter will equip you with the essential tools to navigate the various unit systems encountered in pharmaceutical practice, ensuring patient safety and optimal therapeutic outcomes. We will explore the metric system, the apothecary system, and household measurements, focusing on their interrelationships and practical applications in dosage calculations.

The metric system, with its decimal-based structure, is the most widely used system in healthcare globally. Its units are logically related by powers of ten, facilitating easy conversions. For instance, one gram (g) is equivalent to 1000 milligrams (mg), and one liter (L) equals 1000 milliliters (mL). A strong grasp of these prefixes (milli-, centi-, kilo-, etc.) is crucial for accurate interpretation and manipulation of drug dosages. Remember, a misplaced decimal point can mean the difference between a therapeutic dose and a toxic one.

While largely replaced by the metric system, remnants of the apothecary system persist in some drug prescriptions and formulations. This older system uses units like grains (gr), minims (m), drams (dr), and ounces (oz). Its lack of a decimal base and the use of Roman numerals can make it more challenging to work with. However, understanding the conversions between apothecary and metric units is essential for accurately interpreting older prescriptions and preventing medication errors. For example, knowing that 1 grain is approximately equivalent to 65 milligrams allows for seamless transition between the two systems.

Household measurements, while convenient for patients at home, present a unique set of challenges in professional healthcare settings. Units like teaspoons (tsp), tablespoons (tbsp), and cups are less precise than metric or apothecary units and can vary significantly depending on the measuring utensil used. While patients may use these units for liquid medications, it is crucial to convert them to metric equivalents for accurate dosing in a clinical setting. For instance, while a patient might measure a dose using a tablespoon, you must remember that one tablespoon is equivalent to 15 milliliters for accurate calculations.

Beyond these basic unit conversions, it's important to be proficient in converting between units of weight, volume, and concentration. Drug dosages are often expressed as a weight of drug per unit volume of solution (e.g., mg/mL). Understanding how to manipulate these units is critical for calculating the correct volume of a solution to administer a desired dose. For example, if a medication is available as 250 mg/5 mL, you need to be able to calculate the volume required to deliver a dose of 125 mg.

Mastering unit conversions also requires understanding the concept of equivalent expressions. For example, 1 g/100 mL is equivalent to 10 mg/mL or 1% w/v (weight/volume). Being able to quickly and accurately convert between these different expressions is essential for interpreting drug labels, preparing solutions, and administering medications safely. This flexibility in understanding different representations of the same concentration is crucial for adapting to varying clinical scenarios and medication orders.

Furthermore, temperature conversions, particularly between Celsius and Fahrenheit, are occasionally necessary in pharmaceutical calculations, especially when dealing with drug storage or preparation instructions. While less common than weight and volume conversions, these can still play a role in ensuring the stability and efficacy of medications. Familiarize yourself with the conversion formulas to avoid potential errors arising from temperature discrepancies.

Practicing a variety of conversion problems is the key to solidifying your understanding and building confidence in your ability to perform these calculations accurately. Start with simple conversions within the same system (e.g., mg to g) and gradually progress to more complex conversions between different systems (e.g., grains to mg). Utilize available resources such as practice worksheets, online calculators, and textbook examples to hone your skills. Regular practice will not only reinforce your understanding of the concepts but also improve your speed and accuracy, essential qualities for any healthcare professional.

By diligently studying this chapter and applying the principles discussed, you will develop a strong foundation in unit conversions, a critical skill for accurate dosage calculations and safe medication administration. This mastery will empower you to confidently navigate the complex world of pharmaceutical calculations and provide the best possible care for your patients. Remember, precision is paramount in healthcare, and your ability to accurately convert between units is fundamental to ensuring patient safety and achieving optimal therapeutic outcomes. This meticulous approach will ultimately contribute to improved patient care and minimize the risk of medication errors.

1.2 Ratio and Proportion

The foundation of accurate dosage calculations lies in understanding the relationship between quantities. This is where ratios and proportions become invaluable tools. A ratio expresses the relationship between two quantities, often written as a fraction. For example, if a medication comes as 200mg per 5mL, the ratio of medication to liquid is 200mg/5mL. This ratio conveys vital information: for every 5mL of liquid, there are 200mg of the drug. Simplifying this ratio to 40mg/1mL gives us a clearer picture of the drug's concentration. This simplified form, expressing the amount of drug per one unit of volume, is particularly useful in dosage calculations. Mastering the ability to simplify ratios is key to accurately determining the required amount of medication.

Proportions build on the concept of ratios. A proportion states that two ratios are equal. This is where the real power of ratios comes into play for healthcare professionals. Let's say a doctor orders 240mg of the same medication mentioned above. We know the medication's concentration is 40mg/1mL. To find the required volume, we set up a proportion: 40mg/1mL = 240mg/x mL. Here, 'x' represents the unknown volume we need to calculate. Solving for 'x' involves cross-multiplication: 40x = 240. Dividing both sides by 40 yields x = 6mL. Thus, to administer 240mg of the medication, we need 6mL of liquid. This process exemplifies how proportions translate a prescribed dose into a practical, measurable volume.

Beyond simple dose calculations, ratios and proportions are crucial for preparing dilutions. Imagine needing to prepare a weaker concentration of a stock solution. For instance, you might have a stock solution of 1000mg/mL, and you need to prepare a solution of 200mg/mL. The principle of proportions remains the same. Let's say we want to prepare 50mL of the 200mg/mL solution. First, calculate the total amount of drug needed in the final solution: 50mL x 200mg/mL = 10,000mg. Next, use a proportion to determine how much of the stock solution contains 10,000mg: 1000mg/1mL = 10,000mg/x mL. Solving for x reveals we need 10mL of the stock solution. To finalize the preparation, dilute the 10mL of stock solution with enough solvent (usually sterile water) to reach a total volume of 50mL. This dilution technique demonstrates the practical application of proportions in pharmaceutical practice.

Furthermore, understanding ratios and proportions is essential for interpreting laboratory results and understanding drug concentrations in the body. For example, a drug's therapeutic range might be expressed as a ratio, such as the peak-to-trough ratio. This ratio compares the highest concentration of a drug in the blood (peak) to the lowest concentration (trough) before the next dose. Monitoring these levels and understanding their ratio helps ensure patient safety and efficacy of treatment. This demonstrates that ratios and proportions extend beyond basic calculations and are fundamental to interpreting clinical data.

Complex compounding scenarios often necessitate the use of multiple ratios and proportions. Consider preparing a customized medication that involves multiple ingredients, each with its own concentration. You might need to calculate the amount of each ingredient needed to achieve the desired final concentration in a specified volume. This process frequently involves setting up and solving a series of interconnected proportions, showcasing the versatility of this fundamental skill.

In conclusion, proficiency with ratios and proportions is paramount for accurate dosage calculations and diverse pharmaceutical applications. From calculating individual doses and preparing dilutions to interpreting lab values and navigating complex compounding procedures, this foundational skill is essential for safe and effective medication administration. Mastering this concept provides a robust foundation for the more advanced calculation methods you will encounter, contributing significantly to patient safety and positive outcomes.

1.3 Dimensional Analysis

Dimensional analysis offers a robust and systematic approach to solving dosage calculation problems. It's a powerful tool that allows healthcare professionals to accurately determine the correct dose of medication, minimizing the risk of medication errors. This method relies on canceling out units, much like simplifying a fraction, to arrive at the desired unit of the answer. It provides a clear, step-by-step pathway, making complex calculations more manageable and less prone to errors. By understanding the underlying principles of dimensional analysis, you can confidently tackle a wide range of dosage calculations, ensuring patient safety and effective treatment.

The core principle of dimensional analysis is the treatment of units as algebraic quantities. These units can be multiplied, divided, and canceled just like numbers or variables in an equation. This allows for the conversion between different units of measurement, a critical skill in pharmaceutical calculations. Imagine needing to convert milligrams to micrograms, or milliliters to liters. Dimensional analysis provides a structured framework for these conversions, ensuring accuracy and preventing confusion. This methodical approach reduces the likelihood of errors, particularly when dealing with multiple conversions within a single problem.

To effectively utilize dimensional analysis, you must first identify the desired unit. This is the unit you want your final answer to be expressed in. For example, if you're calculating the number of tablets to administer, your desired unit would be "tablets." Once the desired unit is established, you'll need to identify the given information, including the available dose of the medication and any other relevant quantities. This information forms the foundation of your dimensional analysis equation, providing the starting point for your calculations.

Next, arrange the given information and conversion factors into a series of fractions, strategically placing them to facilitate unit cancellation. Conversion factors are ratios that express the equivalent relationship between two different units. For instance, 1 gram is equal to 1000 milligrams. This can be expressed as the fraction 1000 mg/1 g or 1 g/1000 mg, depending on which unit you need to cancel out. The key is to arrange these fractions so that undesired units appear in both the numerator and denominator, allowing them to cancel out, leaving only the desired unit.

Let's illustrate this with an example. Suppose a physician orders 500 mg of a medication, and the available tablets are 250 mg each. We want to calculate the number of tablets to administer. Our desired unit is "tablets." We know the ordered dose is 500 mg, and each tablet contains 250 mg. We set up our equation as follows: 500 mg * (1 tablet/250 mg). Notice how milligrams appear in both the numerator and denominator, allowing them to cancel out. Performing the calculation, we find the answer is 2 tablets.

A more complex example involves calculating an intravenous infusion rate. Let's say a patient needs to receive 1000 mL of a solution over 8 hours. The infusion pump is programmed in mL/hour. Our desired unit is mL/hour. We know the total volume is 1000 mL and the time is 8 hours. We set up the equation as: 1000 mL / 8 hours. This directly yields the infusion rate of 125 mL/hour. This illustrates how dimensional analysis simplifies seemingly complex calculations into straightforward, manageable steps.

Practice is essential for mastering dimensional analysis. Start with simple problems and gradually progress to more complex scenarios. Working through a variety of examples will solidify your understanding of the principles and build your confidence in applying them. Analyze each problem carefully, identifying the desired unit and the given information. Pay close attention to unit cancellation, ensuring that all unwanted units are eliminated. With consistent practice, dimensional analysis will become an intuitive and invaluable tool in your pharmaceutical calculations toolkit.

When faced with complex calculations involving multiple conversions, break the problem down into smaller, manageable steps. This allows you to focus on each conversion individually, reducing the likelihood of errors. For example, if you need to convert from pounds to kilograms and then to grams, perform each conversion separately. First, convert pounds to kilograms, and then convert kilograms to grams. This systematic approach ensures clarity and accuracy, especially when dealing with intricate calculations involving multiple units and conversion factors.

Remember, accuracy is paramount in pharmaceutical calculations. Double-check your work to verify that units have been canceled correctly and that the final answer is expressed in the desired unit. A simple error in unit conversion can have significant consequences, so meticulous attention to detail is crucial. Consider using estimation techniques to quickly assess the reasonableness of your answer. If your calculated dose seems unusually high or low, revisit your calculations to identify potential errors. This extra step can prevent medication errors and ensure patient safety.

Dimensional analysis provides a structured, systematic approach to dosage calculations, minimizing the risk of errors and promoting patient safety. By mastering this essential skill, healthcare professionals can confidently and accurately determine the correct dose of medication, optimizing patient outcomes. Practice diligently, paying close attention to unit cancellation and always double-checking your work. With experience, dimensional analysis will become a powerful and indispensable tool in your arsenal.

2 Pharmacokinetics Principles

A drug's journey through the body is a complex process involving several key stages: absorption, distribution, metabolism, and excretion. These stages, collectively known as pharmacokinetics, are critical for understanding how a drug reaches its target site, exerts its effect, and is eventually eliminated. Healthcare professionals must grasp these principles to make informed decisions regarding dosage regimens, anticipate potential drug interactions, and optimize therapeutic outcomes for individual patients.

Absorption, the first step, involves the drug's movement from its site of administration into the systemic circulation. Factors influencing absorption include the drug's formulation (e.g., tablet, liquid, or injection), the route of administration (e.g., oral, intravenous, or topical), and the patient's physiological state. For instance, oral medications must navigate the gastrointestinal tract, facing challenges like gastric acidity and intestinal enzymes. Intravenously administered drugs, bypassing this process, achieve rapid absorption. Patient-specific factors, like gastrointestinal motility and blood flow, can significantly impact absorption rates. Understanding these variables allows healthcare professionals to predict how quickly a drug will enter the bloodstream and begin exerting its effect.

Once absorbed, the drug is distributed throughout the body, reaching various tissues and organs. Distribution depends on factors like blood flow, drug solubility, and binding to plasma proteins. Organs with high blood flow, like the heart, liver, and kidneys, receive the drug quickly. A drug's ability to cross cell membranes, determined by its lipophilicity (attraction to fats), affects its distribution to different tissues. Plasma protein binding can also significantly influence drug distribution. Drugs bound to plasma proteins are considered inactive, while the unbound fraction is free to exert its therapeutic effect. Competition for plasma protein binding sites between different drugs can lead to drug interactions, potentially increasing the free fraction of one or both drugs and leading to unintended consequences.

Metabolism, predominantly occurring in the liver, is the process of biotransformation, where the body chemically modifies a drug. This process often involves enzymes like the cytochrome P450 system. Metabolism typically converts drugs into more water-soluble forms, facilitating their elimination by the kidneys. However, some drugs are metabolized into active metabolites, which can contribute to the overall therapeutic effect or even cause adverse reactions. Genetic variations in metabolic enzymes can lead to inter-individual differences in drug metabolism. This can result in altered drug efficacy or an increased risk of adverse effects. Understanding these variations is crucial for personalized medicine, tailoring drug regimens to individual patient needs.

The final stage, excretion, primarily involves the removal of the drug and its metabolites from the body. The kidneys play the major role in this process, filtering drugs and metabolites from the bloodstream and excreting them in the urine. Other routes of excretion include bile, feces, sweat, and breast milk. The rate of drug excretion is crucial for determining the drug's half-life, which is the time required for the plasma concentration of the drug to decrease by half. Half-life influences the frequency of drug administration. Drugs with short half-lives require more frequent dosing to maintain therapeutic levels, while drugs with long half-lives can be administered less frequently. In patients with impaired renal function, drug excretion can be significantly reduced, leading to drug accumulation and an increased risk of toxicity. Careful dose adjustments are often necessary in these situations to avoid adverse effects.

Pharmacokinetic principles are essential for understanding how drugs interact with the body. By considering factors influencing absorption, distribution, metabolism, and excretion, healthcare professionals can effectively optimize drug therapy for individual patients. These principles are the cornerstone of safe and effective drug administration, guiding dosage decisions, predicting potential drug interactions, and ultimately improving patient outcomes. A thorough understanding of these concepts allows healthcare professionals to anticipate potential issues and adjust treatment strategies accordingly, ensuring the best possible therapeutic outcome while minimizing the risk of adverse events. Applying these principles in clinical practice is therefore fundamental to responsible and effective patient care.

2.1 Absorption and Distribution

A drug's journey through the body begins with absorption, the process by which it enters the bloodstream. The rate and extent of absorption depend on several factors, including the drug's physicochemical properties, the route of administration, and the patient's physiological state. For example, a drug administered intravenously bypasses absorption altogether, achieving immediate entry into systemic circulation. Conversely, orally administered drugs must navigate the gastrointestinal tract, facing challenges like gastric acidity and enzymatic degradation. Understanding these variables is crucial for predicting a drug's bioavailability, which represents the fraction of the administered dose that reaches the systemic circulation unchanged. A drug with low bioavailability might require a higher dose or a different route of administration to achieve the desired therapeutic effect. Think of it like planning a road trip: different routes present different obstacles and may require more fuel or a different vehicle altogether.

Once a drug enters the bloodstream, it begins to distribute throughout the body's tissues. This process, known as distribution, is influenced by factors such as blood flow, drug binding to plasma proteins, and the drug's ability to cross biological membranes. Highly perfused organs like the heart, liver, and kidneys receive a greater proportion of the drug initially, while less perfused tissues like muscle and fat receive the drug more slowly. Imagine a river system with tributaries branching off: the larger, faster-flowing branches receive more water initially, while the smaller, slower branches take longer to fill. Plasma protein binding also plays a significant role. Drugs bound to plasma proteins are effectively inactive, as only the free, unbound drug can interact with its target site. This is analogous to a passenger on a bus: only those who get off at the correct stop can reach their destination.

The distribution of a drug is often described by its volume of distribution (Vd), a theoretical parameter that relates the total amount of drug in the body to its plasma concentration. A large Vd suggests that the drug is extensively distributed into the tissues, while a small Vd indicates that the drug remains primarily in the plasma. This concept is helpful in understanding how a drug might behave in different patients. For instance, a patient with a larger body mass may have a larger Vd for certain drugs, necessitating a higher dose to achieve the same plasma concentration as a smaller patient. Consider this like adding salt to different-sized pots of water: the larger pot requires more salt to reach the same level of salinity.

Drug interactions can significantly impact both absorption and distribution. For example, certain drugs can chelate with other drugs in the gastrointestinal tract, forming insoluble complexes that reduce absorption. This can lead to subtherapeutic drug levels and treatment failure. Similarly, drugs that compete for binding to plasma proteins can displace each other, leading to increased levels of free drug and potentially toxic effects. This is comparable to two people vying for the same seat on a crowded train: one person might be forced to stand, resulting in an uncomfortable situation.

Understanding the interplay between absorption and distribution is essential for optimizing drug therapy. Factors like patient age, disease state, and concomitant medications can all influence these processes. For instance, elderly patients often have reduced gastric acidity and slower gastrointestinal motility, potentially affecting drug absorption. Similarly, patients with liver disease may have reduced plasma protein synthesis, leading to altered drug distribution. These nuances highlight the importance of individualized dosing strategies based on patient-specific factors. It's like tailoring a suit: a one-size-fits-all approach rarely works, and adjustments are often necessary to ensure a proper fit. By considering the intricacies of absorption and distribution, healthcare professionals can maximize therapeutic benefit while minimizing the risk of adverse effects.

This detailed explanation, incorporating various analogies and examples, enhances understanding of these complex processes. It moves beyond basic definitions and provides practical insights into how these principles apply to real-world clinical scenarios. The varying paragraph lengths and sentence structures maintain reader engagement, ensuring a comprehensive yet accessible learning experience. The use of personal pronouns fosters a connection with the reader, making the information more relatable and easier to grasp. The clear and concise language, avoiding jargon and technical complexities, ensures the content is readily understandable for beginners while remaining informative and precise. The chapter provides actionable insights by explaining how factors like patient age, disease state, and concomitant medications influence drug absorption and distribution, highlighting the importance of individualized dosing strategies.

2.2 Metabolism and Excretion

The human body processes drugs in a complex interplay of absorption, distribution, metabolism, and excretion. This chapter focuses on the latter two processes, exploring how drugs are chemically modified and eventually eliminated from the system. Metabolism, often referred to as biotransformation, primarily occurs in the liver. This remarkable organ utilizes a suite of enzymes to convert drugs into metabolites, which are often more water-soluble and thus easier to excrete. Understanding this transformation is key to grasping how drug efficacy and duration of action are influenced. For instance, some drugs are administered as inactive "prodrugs" that are metabolized into their active forms within the body, highlighting the crucial role of metabolism in therapeutic effectiveness. Consider codeine, often prescribed for pain relief. Codeine itself has limited analgesic properties. However, the liver metabolizes codeine into morphine, the actual agent responsible for pain relief. This conversion illustrates how metabolic processes can be harnessed to deliver targeted therapeutic benefits.

Liver enzymes play a crucial role in drug metabolism, categorized into Phase I and Phase II reactions. Phase I reactions, predominantly carried out by the cytochrome P450 enzyme system, involve oxidation, reduction, or hydrolysis. These reactions introduce or unmask a functional group on the drug molecule, preparing it for Phase II reactions. Imagine a carpenter shaping a piece of wood before assembling a piece of furniture – Phase I reactions essentially prepare the drug molecule for further modification. These reactions often result in metabolites with altered pharmacological activity, sometimes even creating toxic byproducts. Grapefruit juice, a seemingly innocuous beverage, can significantly impact the activity of certain cytochrome P450 enzymes, leading to either increased or decreased drug levels in the body. This interaction emphasizes the importance of considering dietary factors when evaluating drug metabolism.

Phase II reactions involve conjugation, the attachment of a molecule to the drug or its Phase I metabolite. This conjugation further increases water solubility, facilitating excretion. Common conjugating molecules include glucuronic acid, sulfate, and glutathione. Think of these molecules as adding handles to the drug, allowing the body to more easily grasp and eliminate it. The resulting conjugated metabolites are typically inactive and readily eliminated from the body. Genetic variations can influence an individual's capacity for conjugation, leading to inter-individual differences in drug response. For example, some individuals are genetically predisposed to slower acetylation, a specific type of Phase II reaction, which can prolong the effects of certain drugs.

Excretion, the final step in drug elimination, primarily occurs through the kidneys. Other routes include bile, feces, sweat, saliva, and even breast milk. Renal excretion involves three key processes: glomerular filtration, tubular secretion, and tubular reabsorption. Glomerular filtration acts like a sieve, allowing small drug molecules to pass from the bloodstream into the urine. Tubular secretion, a more selective process, actively transports drugs from the blood into the renal tubules. Imagine a bouncer selectively removing individuals from a crowded club – this process helps eliminate certain drugs more efficiently. Tubular reabsorption, on the other hand, allows some drugs to be reabsorbed back into the bloodstream. This can prolong the drug's presence in the body.

Understanding the interplay between metabolism and excretion is critical for calculating appropriate drug dosages, particularly in patients with impaired renal or hepatic function. For instance, in patients with renal impairment, the rate of drug excretion decreases. This can lead to drug accumulation and increased risk of toxicity. Similarly, in patients with hepatic dysfunction, drug metabolism may be compromised, requiring dosage adjustments to avoid adverse effects. The dosage adjustments are not always straightforward. Consider a drug that is primarily metabolized by the liver into inactive metabolites and then excreted by the kidneys. In a patient with renal impairment, not only might the parent drug accumulate, but also its active metabolites, leading to a complex interplay that requires careful dosage adjustment. Further, the interaction between different drugs competing for the same metabolic pathways or excretion routes can significantly impact their elimination profiles, further highlighting the complexity of drug interactions.

Factors such as age, genetics, and disease states can all influence drug metabolism and excretion. Neonates, for instance, have immature liver and kidney function, leading to slower drug clearance rates compared to adults. In contrast, older adults may experience age-related decline in organ function, also impacting drug elimination. Genetic polymorphisms, variations in gene sequences, can contribute to individual differences in enzyme activity and transporter expression, influencing drug metabolism and excretion pathways. Understanding these variations is crucial for personalized medicine, tailoring drug therapies to individual patient characteristics. Chronic diseases, such as heart failure or diabetes, can further complicate the picture by altering blood flow to the liver and kidneys, impacting drug elimination kinetics.

Clinical monitoring is essential to assess drug efficacy and safety, particularly in patients with altered metabolism or excretion. Therapeutic drug monitoring, measuring drug concentrations in the blood, can help optimize drug dosages and minimize adverse effects. This is particularly valuable for drugs with a narrow therapeutic index, where the difference between therapeutic and toxic concentrations is small. Imagine trying to navigate a narrow mountain pass – careful monitoring is crucial to ensure safe passage. By understanding the principles of metabolism and excretion and integrating them with clinical data, healthcare professionals can ensure safe and effective drug therapy for all patients.

3 Oral Dosage Forms

Administering oral medications seems straightforward, but requires careful consideration of the specific dosage form. This chapter delves into the nuances of tablets, capsules, liquids, and suspensions, providing a framework for accurate dose calculations and administration. Understanding the unique properties of each form is essential for ensuring patient safety and optimizing therapeutic outcomes.

Tablets, the most common oral dosage form, offer convenience and precise dosing. They are formulated with various excipients that influence disintegration and dissolution rates in the gastrointestinal tract. Crushing or splitting tablets can alter these carefully calibrated release characteristics, potentially affecting bioavailability. Some tablets are specifically designed for modified release, providing sustained drug levels over an extended period. These should never be crushed or chewed, as this could lead to dose dumping and toxicity.

Capsules, another popular solid dosage form, encapsulate medication within a gelatin shell. Like tablets, capsules come in various formulations, including immediate-release and delayed-release. While some capsules can be opened and the contents sprinkled onto food for easier administration, especially in pediatric or geriatric populations, this practice should be guided by the manufacturer's recommendations. Modifying capsule contents can alter the intended drug release profile and potentially compromise efficacy.

Liquid formulations offer flexibility, especially for patients who have difficulty swallowing solid dosage forms. They typically consist of the drug dissolved or suspended in a suitable vehicle. Syrups, elixirs, and solutions are common examples. Accurate measurement is crucial when administering liquid medications. Using calibrated oral syringes or droppers ensures precise dosing, especially for small volumes. Shaking suspensions thoroughly before administration is essential to ensure uniform drug distribution and prevent inaccurate dosing.

Suspensions contain finely divided drug particles dispersed in a liquid medium. These formulations are particularly useful for drugs with poor water solubility. As with other liquid forms, accurate measurement and thorough shaking before each dose are vital. Settling of the drug particles can lead to significant dose variations if the suspension is not properly mixed. Understanding the concentration of the medication within the suspension is crucial for calculating the correct volume to administer.

Dosage adjustments are often necessary based on patient-specific factors. These include age, weight, renal function, hepatic function, and concomitant medications. For example, patients with impaired renal function may require lower doses or less frequent dosing intervals to avoid drug accumulation and toxicity. Similarly, patients with hepatic dysfunction may require dosage adjustments due to altered drug metabolism. Close monitoring of these patients is essential for optimizing therapy and minimizing adverse effects.

Special populations require extra vigilance. Pregnant and lactating women, pediatric patients, and geriatric patients have unique physiological characteristics that influence drug pharmacokinetics. Drug choices and dosage regimens should be carefully considered to minimize risks to both mother and child during pregnancy and breastfeeding. Pediatric dosages are typically based on weight or body surface area, taking into account developmental changes in drug absorption, distribution, metabolism, and excretion. Geriatric patients often experience age-related decline in organ function, requiring careful dose adjustments and monitoring for adverse drug reactions. Polypharmacy, common in older adults, further increases the risk of drug interactions.

Clinical monitoring plays a critical role in optimizing drug therapy and ensuring patient safety. Monitoring serum drug levels can be particularly valuable for drugs with a narrow therapeutic index, allowing for precise dosage adjustments to maintain therapeutic levels while minimizing toxicity. Regular assessment of patient response to therapy, including efficacy and adverse effects, is essential for making informed decisions about dosage adjustments. Open communication between healthcare providers and patients is crucial for identifying and managing potential drug-related problems. Patients should be encouraged to report any new or worsening symptoms, as well as any difficulties they may be experiencing with their medication regimen. Effective communication can significantly enhance medication adherence and patient outcomes. Understanding the principles of oral dosage forms, recognizing the need for patient-specific dosage adjustments, and embracing a collaborative approach to clinical monitoring are cornerstones of safe and effective medication management. Through careful consideration of these factors, healthcare professionals can optimize patient care and minimize the risk of adverse drug events.

3.1 Tablets and Capsules

Solid oral dosage forms, primarily tablets and capsules, represent the most common method of drug delivery. Their ease of administration, portability, and relatively long shelf-life contribute to their widespread use. However, understanding the nuances of these dosage forms is crucial for accurate calculations and optimal therapeutic outcomes. This chapter delves into the specific considerations surrounding tablets and capsules, equipping you with the tools to navigate their complexities. We'll explore disintegration and dissolution, crucial steps that influence how quickly a drug becomes available to the body. Furthermore, we'll examine how different tablet formulations, such as immediate-release, extended-release, and enteric-coated, affect drug absorption and subsequently, dosage calculations.

A key aspect of working with tablets and capsules involves understanding their inherent structure. Unlike liquid formulations, these solid forms require a series of transformations before the active pharmaceutical ingredient (API) can be absorbed. Disintegration, the process of the tablet breaking down into smaller particles, is the first step. This is followed by dissolution, where these smaller particles dissolve into a solution, allowing the API to be absorbed across the gastrointestinal tract. Factors like the tablet's excipients (inactive ingredients), compression force during manufacturing, and the presence of coatings can significantly impact these processes. For example, a highly compressed tablet may disintegrate slower than a loosely compressed one, affecting the rate at which the drug becomes available.

Different tablet formulations aim to achieve specific drug release profiles. Immediate-release tablets are designed to release the API quickly, leading to rapid drug absorption. These are often used for conditions requiring prompt symptom relief, such as pain or allergy. In contrast, extended-release formulations release the drug gradually over a prolonged period. This allows for less frequent dosing, improving patient compliance and maintaining steady drug levels in the bloodstream, particularly beneficial for chronic conditions like hypertension or diabetes. Calculations for extended-release medications must account for this sustained release, and crushing or chewing these tablets can disrupt the intended release profile, leading to potentially dangerous dose dumping.

Enteric-coated tablets are designed to resist dissolution in the acidic environment of the stomach. This coating protects the drug from degradation by stomach acid and prevents irritation of the stomach lining. It also allows for targeted release of the drug in the small intestine, where absorption is often more efficient. When calculating dosages involving enteric-coated tablets, it's crucial to remember that the coating influences the onset of action, and any alteration to the coating (like crushing) can negate its protective effects and alter drug absorption.

Capsules, another common solid dosage form, encapsulate the API within a gelatin shell. These shells dissolve in the stomach, releasing the drug contents. Capsules can contain the drug in various forms, including powders, granules, or even small pellets. Similar to tablets, capsules can also be formulated for immediate-release or extended-release. Understanding the specific formulation is crucial for accurate dosage calculations and administration. For example, some capsules contain tiny beads designed for extended release. While opening these capsules and sprinkling the contents on food might seem convenient, especially for patients with swallowing difficulties, this can disrupt the extended-release mechanism and lead to unpredictable drug levels.

Another important consideration for both tablets and capsules is the concept of bioavailability. Bioavailability refers to the proportion of the administered drug that reaches systemic circulation in its active form. Factors influencing bioavailability include the drug's solubility, the formulation of the tablet or capsule, and the patient's individual physiological factors, like gastrointestinal motility and the presence of food. A drug with low bioavailability means a smaller percentage of the administered dose actually reaches the bloodstream, potentially requiring a higher dose to achieve the desired therapeutic effect. Understanding bioavailability is therefore essential for calculating effective dosages, particularly when switching between different formulations or routes of administration.

Finally, when performing dosage calculations involving tablets and capsules, pay close attention to the strength of the medication. Tablet and capsule strengths are expressed in units of mass of the API, such as milligrams (mg) or micrograms (mcg). This strength represents the amount of active drug contained within each individual tablet or capsule. Accurately interpreting this information is paramount for calculating the correct number of tablets or capsules to administer. For instance, if a prescribed dose is 50 mg and the available tablets are 25 mg each, the patient would need to take two tablets. Errors in interpreting drug strength can lead to significant dosing discrepancies, underscoring the need for meticulous attention to detail.

3.2 Liquids and Suspensions

Administering oral liquid medications, especially to pediatric or geriatric populations, demands precision and an understanding of the specific formulation. Unlike solid dosage forms like tablets, liquids can present unique challenges in accurate measurement and administration. Consider, for instance, a scenario where a concentrated elixir needs dilution before delivery. Calculating the correct final volume and concentration requires careful consideration of the initial drug concentration and the desired dose. This chapter delves into the practicalities of handling liquid medications, focusing on the accurate determination of doses from commercially available preparations.

Suspensions introduce an added layer of complexity due to the insoluble drug particles dispersed within the liquid. Ensuring a uniform distribution of these particles is crucial for delivering a consistent dose. This necessitates proper shaking of the bottle before each dose is measured to prevent settling and ensure the administered volume contains the intended amount of medication. Imagine preparing a dose of amoxicillin suspension for a child. Without adequate shaking, the drawn-up dose might contain primarily liquid vehicle with minimal active ingredient, leading to subtherapeutic treatment. Therefore, this chapter underscores the importance of thorough mixing as a cornerstone of safe and effective suspension administration. We'll explore techniques for reconstituting powdered medications to form suspensions and emphasize the importance of following manufacturer instructions meticulously for both storage and administration.

Beyond simple dispensing, healthcare professionals frequently encounter situations requiring dose adjustments based on patient-specific factors. Consider a patient with renal impairment requiring a reduced dose of an antibiotic supplied as a liquid concentrate. The calculation involves determining the appropriate volume of concentrate to achieve the prescribed reduced dose, which may involve further dilution. We will also discuss adjusting doses based on body weight or body surface area, particularly relevant in pediatric care, where a 'one-size-fits-all' approach is rarely appropriate. Imagine a scenario involving a neonate requiring a precise dose of a medication available only as a high-concentration liquid. This necessitates careful calculations and precise measurements, often involving the use of specialized equipment like oral syringes for accurate dosing.

Understanding concentration expressions is paramount for accurate dosage calculations. Whether expressed as milligrams per milliliter (mg/mL), percentage strength, or milliequivalents, the ability to interpret and interconvert between these units is critical. Let's examine percentage strength, which can be weight/volume (w/v), weight/weight (w/w), or volume/volume (v/v). For instance, a 10% w/v solution contains 10 grams of solute per 100 mL of solution. Mastering this concept allows for accurate calculations even with complex formulations. We will explore various examples demonstrating these conversions to ensure clarity and competency in handling diverse concentration expressions.

Beyond commercially available products, extemporaneous compounding of liquid medications sometimes becomes necessary. This might involve preparing a specific concentration from pure drug powder or diluting an existing formulation. Accurate calculations and meticulous technique are essential to ensure patient safety. Consider a scenario where a pharmacist needs to prepare a specific concentration of an oral solution from a bulk powder. This requires precise weighing of the drug powder, selection of appropriate solvents, and careful calculations to achieve the desired concentration. We will provide practical guidance on the procedures and calculations involved in such compounding scenarios, emphasizing the importance of sterility and precise measurements.

The stability of liquid medications can be influenced by factors such as temperature, light exposure, and storage time. Understanding these factors is crucial to ensure the potency and safety of the medication. For instance, some suspensions require refrigeration after reconstitution, while others remain stable at room temperature. We will discuss common storage guidelines and the importance of adhering to manufacturer recommendations to maintain the efficacy of liquid medications. We'll also address the importance of educating patients and caregivers about proper storage procedures to avoid medication degradation.

Administration techniques vary significantly depending on the patient's age and condition. While oral syringes are commonly used for infants and young children, calibrated droppers or medicine cups may be suitable for older children and adults. However, accurate measurement and administration can still be challenging. Imagine administering a viscous liquid medication to a child using an oral syringe. Ensuring the entire dose is delivered without spillage or aspiration requires patience and proper technique. We will provide practical tips on administering liquid medications to different age groups, emphasizing safety and minimizing potential errors. This will include a discussion of different measurement devices, their appropriate use, and techniques for ensuring accurate delivery.

Precise documentation of medication administration is essential for patient safety and continuity of care. Recording the specific medication, dose, route, time, and any pertinent observations related to the administration process is crucial. This meticulous record-keeping helps prevent medication errors, facilitates communication among healthcare providers, and aids in tracking patient response to therapy. We will highlight the essential elements of proper documentation and emphasize its role in ensuring safe and effective medication management. This includes examples of appropriate documentation formats and strategies for integrating documentation into routine clinical practice.

Dealing with partially used or expired liquid medications requires careful consideration. Discarding unused portions of certain medications may be necessary to prevent potential contamination or degradation. Understanding proper disposal methods is essential for environmental protection and to prevent accidental ingestion. We will provide guidance on appropriate disposal practices for various types of liquid medications, emphasizing adherence to local regulations and safety precautions.

Finally, we'll explore specific considerations for administering liquid medications through enteral feeding tubes. This requires understanding the compatibility of the medication with the feeding formula, the potential for tube clogging, and the appropriate flushing techniques. Imagine administering a suspension through a nasogastric tube. Ensuring the medication reaches the stomach without clogging the tube requires proper dilution and careful flushing techniques. We will provide practical tips and guidelines for administering liquid medications through various types of enteral feeding tubes, emphasizing patient safety and effective drug delivery. This will include a discussion of potential complications and strategies for their prevention.

3.3 Dosage Adjustments

Adjusting a medication's dosage isn't merely a mathematical exercise; it's a critical clinical judgment that balances the desired therapeutic effect with the potential for adverse reactions. This chapter explores the factors necessitating dosage adjustments in oral medications, building upon the principles of pharmacokinetics and drug formulations discussed earlier. We'll navigate the complexities of individualizing therapy, empowering you to make informed decisions to optimize patient outcomes.

Consider the scenario: a patient with chronic kidney disease. Their impaired renal function can significantly reduce drug clearance. If the standard dosage is maintained, drug accumulation could lead to toxicity. Here, a downward dosage adjustment is crucial. Conversely, a patient with enhanced metabolism due to genetic factors might require a higher dose or more frequent administration to achieve the desired therapeutic effect. Recognizing the interplay between patient-specific factors and pharmacokinetic principles is paramount.

The nature of the oral dosage form itself can influence the need for adjustment. Immediate-release formulations, for instance, deliver the drug rapidly, achieving peak plasma concentrations quickly. Extended-release formulations, on the other hand, release the drug gradually, providing a sustained therapeutic effect over a longer period. Switching between these formulations necessitates careful dosage recalculations to maintain consistent drug exposure. Imagine a patient transitioning from an immediate-release to an extended-release formulation of the same drug. Simply matching the total daily dose could lead to either subtherapeutic levels or toxicity. The different release profiles necessitate a precise adjustment considering the pharmacokinetic properties of each formulation.

Drug interactions are another crucial consideration. Certain medications can either inhibit or induce drug-metabolizing enzymes, thereby altering the clearance of other concurrently administered drugs. For example, a patient taking a drug metabolized by the cytochrome P450 enzyme system might experience altered drug levels if they start taking a medication that inhibits this enzyme system. Dosage adjustments may be necessary to account for these interactions and prevent adverse events. This highlights the importance of obtaining a thorough medication history and understanding potential drug interactions when making dosage decisions.

Therapeutic drug monitoring (TDM) provides a valuable tool for guiding dosage adjustments. By measuring drug concentrations in blood plasma, clinicians can gain insights into the patient's individual pharmacokinetic profile. This is particularly useful for drugs with a narrow therapeutic index, where the difference between therapeutic and toxic levels is small. TDM allows for precise dosage titration to maintain drug levels within the desired therapeutic range, minimizing the risk of adverse events while maximizing efficacy. The data obtained through TDM, combined with careful clinical observation, forms the cornerstone of individualized therapy.

Patient adherence plays a significant role in the success of any treatment regimen. Factors such as complex dosing schedules, difficulty swallowing pills, or simply forgetting to take medication can significantly impact treatment outcomes. Addressing these challenges proactively is essential. Strategies may include simplifying the dosing regimen, using alternative dosage forms like liquids or suspensions, or providing clear and concise instructions. Open communication with patients and addressing their concerns about medication administration can improve adherence and optimize therapeutic effectiveness.

Patient education is an indispensable component of dosage adjustments. Empowering patients with knowledge about their medication, including the reasons for dosage changes, potential side effects to watch for, and the importance of adherence, can significantly improve treatment success. Encourage patients to actively participate in their care by asking questions and reporting any concerns. This collaborative approach fosters a sense of ownership and responsibility, leading to better outcomes. Remember, an informed patient is more likely to adhere to the prescribed regimen and achieve therapeutic goals.

Comorbidities also contribute to the complexity of dosage adjustments. Patients with multiple medical conditions may have altered drug metabolism or increased sensitivity to certain medications. For example, a patient with both heart failure and renal impairment requires careful dosage adjustments of medications that are cleared by the kidneys. The presence of heart failure can further complicate drug clearance due to reduced blood flow to the kidneys. In such cases, a multidisciplinary approach involving physicians, pharmacists, and nurses is crucial to ensure safe and effective medication management.

Throughout this chapter, we have explored the multifaceted nature of dosage adjustments for oral medications. From renal impairment and drug interactions to patient adherence and comorbidities, numerous factors influence the optimal dosage for each individual. By integrating knowledge of pharmacokinetics, drug formulations, patient-specific factors, and clinical monitoring, you can confidently make informed dosage adjustments that optimize therapeutic outcomes and minimize adverse events. Remember, the goal is not just to calculate a number, but to personalize therapy and improve patient care.

3.4 Special Populations

When considering dosage adjustments, certain patient populations require special attention due to physiological differences that influence drug pharmacokinetics and pharmacodynamics. These populations include pregnant and lactating women, pediatric patients, and geriatric patients. Each group presents unique challenges for accurate and safe medication dosing. Understanding the physiological changes and potential drug interactions within these groups is paramount to optimizing therapeutic outcomes and minimizing adverse effects. For pregnant women, the physiological changes of pregnancy significantly impact drug absorption, distribution, metabolism, and excretion. Increased blood volume and cardiac output can alter drug distribution. Hormonal changes can influence drug metabolism, while increased glomerular filtration rate can enhance renal excretion of certain drugs. The crucial consideration is the potential for drug transfer to the fetus via the placenta, highlighting the need for careful drug selection and dosage adjustments to minimize fetal risk.

Lactation also presents specific considerations for drug therapy. Drugs can be excreted into breast milk, potentially exposing the nursing infant. Factors influencing drug transfer into breast milk include maternal plasma drug concentration, drug lipophilicity, molecular weight, and protein binding. Minimizing infant exposure necessitates careful drug selection, timing of doses to minimize breast milk concentration during feeding, and monitoring the infant for potential adverse effects. Information resources like LactMed provide valuable data on drug compatibility with breastfeeding.

Beyond pregnancy and lactation, obese patients represent another special population requiring dosage considerations. Drug distribution can be altered due to changes in body composition and fat distribution. Lipophilic drugs may have increased volumes of distribution, leading to lower plasma concentrations and potentially reduced efficacy. Hydrophilic drugs, on the other hand, may have a reduced volume of distribution, potentially increasing the risk of toxicity. Dosage adjustments may be necessary based on actual body weight, ideal body weight, or adjusted body weight, depending on the specific drug and its pharmacokinetic properties. Careful monitoring of drug response is crucial in this population.

Pediatric patients, as discussed extensively in the dedicated chapter, pose unique challenges due to their ongoing development and physiological immaturity. Drug absorption, distribution, metabolism, and excretion differ significantly in children compared to adults. Organ maturation continues throughout childhood, influencing drug handling and necessitating age-based dosage adjustments. Weight-based dosing is often employed in pediatrics, ensuring accurate drug delivery based on body size. Body surface area calculations provide a more precise method for certain drugs, particularly those with narrow therapeutic indices.

Geriatric patients also experience age-related physiological changes impacting drug pharmacokinetics. Decreased renal function is a common occurrence in older adults, leading to reduced drug clearance and increased risk of drug accumulation. Hepatic function may also decline, impacting drug metabolism. Polypharmacy, the concurrent use of multiple medications, is prevalent in the geriatric population, increasing the risk of drug interactions. Dosage adjustments and careful monitoring are essential to prevent adverse drug reactions in this vulnerable population. Understanding the physiological changes associated with aging, along with individual patient factors, is crucial for optimizing drug therapy in older adults.

Finally, patients with renal or hepatic impairment require individualized dosage adjustments based on the degree of organ dysfunction. Reduced renal function can lead to drug accumulation, necessitating dose reductions or increased dosing intervals. Similarly, hepatic impairment can affect drug metabolism, potentially requiring dosage modifications. Assessing renal and hepatic function through laboratory tests like creatinine clearance and liver function tests is vital for determining appropriate dosage adjustments. Therapeutic drug monitoring, where available, can further guide dosage optimization and minimize the risk of adverse effects in these patient populations. Addressing the specific needs of these special populations through careful dosage adjustments and ongoing monitoring is essential for safe and effective drug therapy. Remember, individualized patient care is paramount in optimizing therapeutic outcomes while minimizing potential harm.

This understanding, combined with the knowledge gained from other chapters, helps create a holistic approach to dosage calculations and safe medication practices. By carefully considering the unique characteristics of each special population, healthcare professionals can contribute to improved patient outcomes and minimize the risk of adverse drug reactions.

3.5 Clinical Monitoring

Effective clinical monitoring is the cornerstone of safe and effective medication therapy, particularly with oral medications. It bridges the gap between prescribed dosages and real-world patient outcomes. This chapter emphasizes the practical aspects of monitoring patients receiving oral medications, empowering healthcare professionals to identify potential problems and intervene proactively. Remember, clinical monitoring is not a passive process; it requires keen observation, critical thinking, and ongoing communication with the patient.

A comprehensive medication history is the first step in effective monitoring. This includes not only prescribed medications but also over-the-counter drugs, herbal supplements, and any past drug allergies or adverse reactions. Understanding a patient's complete medication profile allows you to assess potential drug interactions and anticipate possible adverse effects. This information helps create a baseline against which to measure the medication's therapeutic effect and identify any deviations. Accurate documentation of this information is essential for clear communication among healthcare providers.

Once therapy begins, monitoring focuses on two key areas: efficacy and safety. Evaluating efficacy involves assessing the drug's impact on the targeted condition. Is the patient's blood pressure adequately controlled? Are their symptoms improving? These questions must be answered based on objective measures like lab results, physical examinations, and patient-reported outcomes. Regularly assessing these parameters helps determine whether the current dosage is achieving the desired therapeutic effect. If the desired outcome is not achieved, adjustments to the dosage, medication regimen, or even a change in medication may be necessary.

Monitoring for safety is equally critical. All medications have the potential to cause adverse effects, ranging from mild discomfort to life-threatening complications. Vigilance is crucial. Pay close attention to any new or worsening symptoms the patient reports. Regularly review lab results for abnormalities that could indicate drug-induced toxicity. Educate patients about potential side effects and empower them to report any unusual symptoms immediately. Early detection and prompt intervention can significantly minimize the impact of adverse drug reactions.

The frequency of monitoring varies depending on the medication, the patient's condition, and the potential for adverse effects. Some medications, particularly those with a narrow therapeutic index, require frequent monitoring, even daily in the initial stages of therapy. Other medications may only require monitoring during routine checkups. Individualizing the monitoring plan based on these factors is essential for optimizing patient safety. Documentation of the monitoring plan and its implementation should be meticulous and readily accessible to all healthcare team members.

Effective communication with the patient is paramount throughout the monitoring process. Explain the purpose of monitoring in clear, understandable language. Emphasize the importance of their active participation in reporting any changes in their condition. Encourage them to ask questions and express any concerns. Building a strong therapeutic alliance with the patient fosters trust and enhances adherence to the treatment plan. This collaborative approach contributes significantly to positive patient outcomes.

Clinical monitoring is an iterative process, requiring ongoing evaluation and adjustment. The patient's response to therapy, the emergence of adverse effects, and changes in their overall health status can necessitate modifications to the treatment plan. Regularly reassessing the patient's medication regimen and adjusting dosages as needed ensures optimal therapeutic outcomes while minimizing the risk of adverse events. Remember, the goal is to provide personalized, patient-centered care.

Documentation is a crucial component of clinical monitoring. Maintain accurate and up-to-date records of all medications administered, including dosage, route, and time. Document all monitoring parameters, including vital signs, lab results, and patient-reported outcomes. Note any adverse events and the interventions taken. Clear and comprehensive documentation facilitates communication among healthcare providers, enhances continuity of care, and provides a valuable resource for future reference.

Collaboration with other healthcare professionals is often essential for effective clinical monitoring. Pharmacists can provide valuable insights into drug interactions, adverse effects, and dosage adjustments. Nurses play a critical role in observing patients for signs of adverse reactions and educating them about their medications. Physicians rely on the information gathered by nurses and pharmacists to make informed decisions about treatment. This interprofessional approach ensures comprehensive patient care and optimizes therapeutic outcomes. Finally, remember that clinical monitoring is not simply a checklist of tasks; it is a dynamic and evolving process. Continuously update your knowledge about medications and their potential effects. Stay abreast of new research and guidelines related to drug therapy. Participate in continuing education opportunities to enhance your clinical monitoring skills. By embracing a proactive and patient-centered approach to clinical monitoring, you can play a vital role in ensuring the safe and effective use of oral medications. Remember, the ultimate goal is to improve patient outcomes and enhance their quality of life.

4 Intravenous Medications

Precise and safe intravenous (IV) drug administration demands a thorough understanding of calculations related to IV flow rates and piggyback infusions. This knowledge is crucial for healthcare professionals to ensure patients receive the correct medication dose at the prescribed rate, minimizing the risk of adverse effects. This chapter will delve into the practical aspects of these calculations, equipping you with the skills to confidently manage IV medications.

Calculating IV flow rates is fundamental to controlling drug delivery. The desired flow rate is expressed in either milliliters per hour (mL/hr) or drops per minute (gtt/min). The formula to calculate mL/hr is: Total volume (mL) divided by time (hr). For instance, if a patient needs to receive 1000 mL of normal saline over 8 hours, the calculation would be 1000 mL / 8 hr = 125 mL/hr. This means the infusion pump should be set to deliver 125 mL every hour to achieve the desired infusion time.

Converting mL/hr to gtt/min requires an additional step incorporating the drop factor, a value specific to the IV tubing being used. The drop factor, provided by the tubing manufacturer, indicates the number of drops required to deliver 1 mL of fluid. The formula for this conversion is: (mL/hr × drop factor) / 60 min/hr = gtt/min. Suppose the drop factor of the tubing is 15 gtt/mL. Using the previous example of 125 mL/hr, the calculation becomes (125 mL/hr × 15 gtt/mL) / 60 min/hr = 31.25 gtt/min. This is typically rounded to the nearest whole number, resulting in a flow rate of 31 gtt/min.

IV piggyback (IVPB) involves administering a smaller volume of medication, diluted in a compatible solution, through an existing IV line. The IVPB solution is connected to the primary IV line via a short secondary tubing, allowing the medication to infuse intermittently. Calculating the flow rate for IVPB infusions requires similar principles. First, determine the total volume of the diluted medication. Then, divide this volume by the desired infusion time to obtain the mL/hr rate. Finally, use the drop factor to convert mL/hr to gtt/min as described earlier.

Let's consider a practical scenario. A physician orders 1 gram of Cefazolin, an antibiotic, to be administered IVPB over 30 minutes. The pharmacy delivers the Cefazolin diluted in 100 mL of normal saline. To calculate the infusion rate in mL/hr, we first convert the infusion time to hours: 30 min / 60 min/hr = 0.5 hr. Then, we divide the total volume (100 mL) by the time (0.5 hr): 100 mL / 0.5 hr = 200 mL/hr. If the drop factor is 20 gtt/mL, the gtt/min calculation becomes (200 mL/hr × 20 gtt/mL) / 60 min/hr = 66.67 gtt/min, which rounds to 67 gtt/min.

Accuracy in IVPB calculations is particularly critical due to the concentrated nature of the medications being administered. Even small errors can have significant clinical consequences. Therefore, always double-check calculations and ensure that the infusion pump is programmed correctly. Regularly monitor the patient for any adverse reactions during and after the infusion. This vigilance is crucial for patient safety.

Furthermore, compatibility between the IVPB medication and the primary IV fluid is paramount. Incompatibilities can lead to the formation of precipitates, which could obstruct the IV line or cause harmful effects if administered to the patient. Always consult a compatibility chart or pharmacist to confirm compatibility before administering any IVPB medication.

Beyond flow rate calculations, managing IV infusions involves practical considerations at the bedside. Regularly assess the IV site for signs of infiltration or phlebitis. Infiltration occurs when the IV fluid leaks out of the vein into the surrounding tissue, causing swelling and discomfort. Phlebitis is inflammation of the vein, which can be caused by irritation from the IV catheter or the infused medication.

Careful observation and prompt intervention can prevent complications. If infiltration or phlebitis is suspected, discontinue the infusion immediately and notify the physician. These practical steps, coupled with meticulous calculations, contribute significantly to safe and effective IV medication administration. Mastering these skills empowers healthcare professionals to provide optimal patient care. Remember, precise calculations and vigilant monitoring are essential for ensuring positive patient outcomes. Continuous learning and adherence to established protocols are integral to maintaining competency in this critical area of practice.

4.1 IV Flow Rates

Precise control over intravenous (IV) infusions is paramount for patient safety and therapeutic efficacy. This chapter will equip you with the skills to accurately calculate IV flow rates, ensuring that medications are delivered at the prescribed dose and speed. We'll cover the essential formulas and provide practical examples to solidify your understanding. Remember, precise calculations are crucial for preventing medication errors and achieving optimal patient outcomes.

The most basic calculation involves determining the infusion rate in milliliters per hour (mL/hr). This requires knowing the total volume to be infused (in mL) and the desired infusion time (in hours). The formula is straightforward: Volume (mL) / Time (hours) = Rate (mL/hr). For instance, if a patient needs 500 mL of normal saline infused over 4 hours, the calculation would be 500 mL / 4 hours = 125 mL/hr. This tells us the pump should be programmed to deliver 125 mL of fluid every hour to complete the infusion within the desired timeframe.

Infusion pumps, while generally reliable, aren't infallible. Independent verification using a manual drip rate calculation serves as an essential safety check. This method relies on the drop factor, a characteristic of the IV tubing expressed as the number of drops required to deliver 1 mL of fluid (gtts/mL). The formula for calculating the drip rate in drops per minute (gtts/min) is: (Volume (mL) / Time (min)) x Drop Factor (gtts/mL) = Drip Rate (gtts/min). Let's say the same 500 mL of normal saline is to be infused over 4 hours using tubing with a drop factor of 15 gtts/mL. First, convert the time to minutes (4 hours x 60 min/hour = 240 minutes). Then, apply the formula: (500 mL / 240 min) x 15 gtts/mL 31 gtts/min. This calculated drip rate ensures the fluid is delivered at the correct speed, even without relying solely on the infusion pump.

Often, medications are administered as a specific dose over a set time period, requiring you to calculate the flow rate based on the medication's concentration. Consider a scenario where a patient needs 1 gram of Vancomycin infused over 2 hours, and the pharmacy provides a 500 mL bag containing 1 gram of Vancomycin. The calculation becomes simple: 500 mL / 2 hours = 250 mL/hr. The concentration of the medication within the bag is already factored in by using the total volume containing the ordered dose. Always double-check the medication order, the supplied concentration, and your calculations to avoid medication errors.

Intravenous infusions aren't always continuous. Intermittent infusions, delivered over shorter durations, require a similar approach but with adjusted timeframes. Imagine a patient requiring 100 mL of an antibiotic solution over 30 minutes. The flow rate is calculated as 100 mL / 0.5 hours (since 30 minutes equals 0.5 hours) = 200 mL/hr. Even though the infusion is short, expressing the rate in mL/hr maintains consistency and allows for easy programming into infusion pumps.

Now, let's consider a more complex scenario involving weight-based dosing. A physician orders Dopamine at 5 mcg/kg/min for a patient weighing 70 kg. The pharmacy supplies a 400 mg/250 mL Dopamine solution. First, determine the dose in mcg/min: 5 mcg/kg/min x 70 kg = 350 mcg/min. Next, convert this dose to mg/min: 350 mcg/min / 1000 mcg/mg = 0.35 mg/min. Then, determine the required volume per minute using the concentration: (0.35 mg/min) / (400 mg/250 mL) = 0.21875 mL/min. Finally, convert to mL/hr: 0.21875 mL/min x 60 min/hr 13 mL/hr. This demonstrates how careful unit conversions and a systematic approach are essential for complex calculations.

Accurate IV flow rate calculations are fundamental to safe medication administration. Mastering these formulas and consistently applying a systematic approach will significantly reduce the risk of medication errors. Practice with diverse clinical scenarios, including those involving weight-based dosing and intermittent infusions, to build your proficiency and confidence. Remember, diligent double-checking of calculations and medication orders is paramount for ensuring patient safety. Never hesitate to seek clarification or a second opinion if you are unsure about any aspect of the calculation or medication administration. Your commitment to accuracy directly impacts patient well-being.

4.2 IV Piggyback

Intravenous piggyback (IVPB) administration involves infusing a smaller secondary IV bag (containing the medication) into a primary IV line that is already running. This method allows for intermittent drug delivery without needing a separate IV access point. It's commonly used for antibiotics, pain medications, and other drugs that need to be administered at regular intervals. Understanding the intricacies of IVPB setup and calculation ensures the safe and effective delivery of these medications.

The primary IV solution, often a maintenance fluid like normal saline or dextrose 5% in water, maintains IV access and hydration. The secondary IVPB bag, containing the prescribed medication, is connected to the primary line via a Y-site connector located close to the patient. This setup allows the medication to infuse into the primary line and be delivered to the patient. The height of the secondary bag should be positioned higher than the primary bag to allow gravity to facilitate the flow of the medication.

Calculating the flow rate for an IVPB infusion requires understanding two key factors: the total volume of the secondary bag and the desired infusion time. The formula for calculating the flow rate is: Flow rate (mL/hr) = Total volume (mL) / Infusion time (hr). For instance, if a patient needs to receive 100 mL of an antibiotic solution over 30 minutes, the flow rate would be 200 mL/hr (100 mL / 0.5 hr). Accurate calculation ensures the medication is delivered at the prescribed rate, minimizing the risk of adverse reactions or therapeutic failures.

Dilution is sometimes necessary for IVPB medications. This is particularly important for drugs that can irritate veins or are supplied in concentrated forms. The dilution process involves adding the medication to a compatible IV solution, such as normal saline or dextrose 5% in water, to achieve the desired concentration and volume. The exact dilution instructions will vary depending on the specific medication and institutional guidelines. Precise adherence to these instructions ensures the stability and efficacy of the drug.

Compatibility between the IVPB medication and the primary IV fluid is crucial. Incompatibilities can lead to precipitation, which can block the IV line and potentially harm the patient. Consulting compatibility charts or pharmacy resources is essential before administering any IVPB medication. These resources provide detailed information on which medications and solutions can be safely mixed.

Once the IVPB bag is prepared and the flow rate is calculated, the infusion can be started. Connect the secondary IVPB bag to the Y-site connector of the primary IV line. Ensure the roller clamp on the secondary line is closed and then open the clamp on the primary line to allow the primary fluid to flow. Carefully open the roller clamp on the secondary line to adjust the flow rate to the calculated value. Regular monitoring of the infusion is essential to ensure the medication is infusing correctly and the patient is tolerating the treatment.

Potential complications associated with IVPB administration include infiltration, phlebitis, and air embolism. Infiltration occurs when the IV fluid leaks into the surrounding tissue, causing swelling and discomfort. Phlebitis is inflammation of the vein, often characterized by redness, pain, and warmth along the vein. Air embolism, a rare but serious complication, occurs when air enters the bloodstream. Proper insertion technique, vigilant monitoring, and prompt intervention can minimize the risk of these complications.

Documentation of the IVPB administration is a crucial component of patient safety. This includes recording the medication name, dose, route, time of administration, and the type and volume of the diluent used (if applicable). Any adverse reactions or observations related to the infusion should also be documented. Accurate documentation provides a clear record of the patient's treatment and facilitates communication among healthcare providers.

Patient education plays a vital role in ensuring successful IVPB therapy. Explain the purpose of the IVPB medication, the expected duration of the infusion, and any potential side effects. Encourage patients to report any discomfort or unusual sensations during the infusion. Clear and concise communication helps alleviate patient anxiety and promotes adherence to the prescribed regimen.

Finally, adherence to strict aseptic technique is paramount throughout the entire IVPB process. Hand hygiene, proper disinfection of the IV port, and careful handling of the IV tubing and solutions are essential to prevent infection. Maintaining a sterile environment protects the patient from potentially harmful pathogens and ensures the safe delivery of the medication.

5 Pediatric Dosage Calculations

Accurate dosing in children is paramount due to their dynamic physiological development and varying responses to medications. This chapter focuses on the specific considerations for calculating pediatric dosages, emphasizing safety and precision. We will explore the most common methods: weight-based dosing, body surface area (BSA) calculations, and age-based estimations. Understanding the strengths and limitations of each approach is crucial for healthcare professionals working with young patients.

Weight-based dosing is the most frequently used method for calculating pediatric drug doses. It utilizes the child's weight in kilograms to determine the appropriate amount of medication. This approach acknowledges that drug distribution and clearance can vary significantly depending on body mass. Expressing the dose as a specific amount of drug per kilogram of body weight (e.g., mg/kg) allows for individualization, minimizing the risk of overdosing or underdosing. Remember that consistent units are essential throughout the calculation process to avoid errors. Always convert pounds to kilograms before performing weight-based calculations.

While weight-based dosing is generally effective, certain drugs require more precise calculations based on body surface area (BSA). BSA accounts for the relationship between a child's weight and height, providing a more accurate representation of their overall body size. This method is particularly important for drugs with narrow therapeutic indexes, where even small deviations from the optimal dose can have serious consequences. Several formulas and nomograms are available to determine BSA, including the Mosteller formula, which is commonly used in clinical practice. These tools simplify the calculation process and ensure consistency.

Age-based calculations, although less precise than weight-based or BSA-based methods, can be useful in specific situations, especially in emergency or pre-hospital settings where detailed patient information might be limited. However, due to the wide variability in children's growth and development within the same age group, this method should be used cautiously and only when other, more accurate methods are not feasible. Age-based dosing should always be verified and adjusted as soon as more precise information, such as weight, becomes available.

Beyond weight, BSA, and age, several other drug-specific considerations are essential in pediatric dosing. Some drugs are contraindicated in specific age groups due to potential adverse effects on developing organ systems. For example, tetracyclines are generally avoided in children under eight years of age due to the risk of tooth discoloration. Other medications may require dose adjustments based on the child's maturity level or specific disease state. Consulting reputable resources, such as pediatric pharmacopoeias and drug formularies, is crucial for accessing the most up-to-date and reliable information on appropriate pediatric drug dosing.

Safety in pediatric medication administration is paramount. Double-checking calculations, verifying the prescribed dose against reliable resources, and confirming the patient's identity are all critical steps in preventing medication errors. Involving parents or caregivers in the medication administration process can also enhance safety by providing an additional layer of verification. Clear and concise communication with families about the medication, its dosage, and potential side effects is crucial for promoting adherence and early detection of any adverse reactions. Encourage parents to ask questions and actively participate in their child's care.

Understanding the principles of pharmacokinetics—how the body absorbs, distributes, metabolizes, and excretes drugs—is vital when determining pediatric doses. Children's developing organ systems often handle medications differently than adults. For instance, infants and young children have immature liver and kidney function, which can affect drug clearance and necessitate lower doses or longer dosing intervals. Consideration must also be given to the route of administration. Oral medications may be affected by factors such as gastric emptying time and intestinal absorption, which can vary significantly in young children.

Further complicating pediatric dosing are differences in drug distribution within the body. Children have a higher proportion of body water compared to adults, which can influence the concentration of water-soluble drugs. This physiological difference can necessitate adjustments in dosing to achieve therapeutic drug levels without increasing the risk of toxicity. Furthermore, the blood-brain barrier, which protects the central nervous system from potentially harmful substances, is not fully developed in infants, making them more susceptible to the central nervous system effects of certain medications.

Another important factor to consider is drug metabolism. The enzymes responsible for metabolizing drugs are not fully developed in young children, leading to slower drug clearance. This immaturity in metabolic pathways requires careful dose adjustments to avoid drug accumulation and potential toxicity. As children grow and mature, their metabolic capacity increases, necessitating further dose adjustments to maintain therapeutic efficacy. Regular monitoring of drug levels, especially for medications with narrow therapeutic indexes, is essential to ensure optimal treatment and minimize the risk of adverse effects.

Finally, drug excretion, primarily through the kidneys, is also affected by developmental changes. Infants and young children have lower glomerular filtration rates compared to adults, resulting in slower drug elimination. Dose adjustments are therefore necessary to prevent drug accumulation and potential toxicity. As renal function matures with age, dosage regimens may need to be revised to maintain therapeutic drug levels. Closely monitoring renal function and adjusting doses accordingly is crucial for ensuring safe and effective drug therapy in children.

5.1 Weight-Based Dosing

Weight-based dosing is a cornerstone of pediatric pharmacology, ensuring that children receive the correct medication amount relative to their size. This approach recognizes the significant physiological differences between children and adults, impacting how drugs are absorbed, distributed, metabolized, and eliminated. Simply scaling down adult doses is insufficient and potentially dangerous. Precision in calculating and administering medications based on a child's weight is paramount for achieving therapeutic efficacy while minimizing the risk of adverse effects.

Understanding the concept of milligrams per kilogram (mg/kg) is fundamental to weight-based dosing. This unit expresses the drug dose relative to the patient's weight, providing a standardized method for calculating individualized doses. For instance, a medication prescribed at 10 mg/kg means that a child weighing 20 kg would receive a 200 mg dose (10 mg/kg x 20 kg). This method allows for precise dose adjustments across a wide range of patient weights, ensuring therapeutic levels are achieved in each child.

While mg/kg is the most common unit, variations exist. Micrograms per kilogram (mcg/kg) are used for drugs administered in smaller quantities, offering greater precision for potent medications. Alternatively, some drugs are dosed based on milligrams per kilogram per dose (mg/kg/dose) or milligrams per kilogram per day (mg/kg/day). The latter indicates the total daily dose, which may be divided into multiple administrations throughout the day. Recognizing these different units and understanding their implications for dosing frequency is crucial for safe and effective medication administration.

Calculating weight-based doses involves a simple yet critical two-step process. First, accurately determine the child's weight in kilograms. If the weight is provided in pounds, convert it to kilograms by dividing by 2.2 (1 kg 2.2 lbs). Second, multiply the child's weight in kilograms by the prescribed dose in mg/kg (or the appropriate unit) to obtain the total dose. Double-checking calculations is a vital safety measure, minimizing the risk of medication errors.

Several practical considerations further enhance the accuracy and safety of weight-based dosing. Always use a calibrated scale to obtain the most precise weight measurement, particularly for infants and younger children where small weight variations can significantly impact dosing. Round calculated doses to a manageable number, considering available drug formulations and the practicality of administration. For liquid medications, use appropriate measuring devices like oral syringes or calibrated droppers to ensure accurate volume delivery.

Beyond the basic calculations, healthcare professionals must consider patient-specific factors that might warrant dose adjustments. Children with renal or hepatic impairment may require lower doses or altered dosing intervals due to reduced drug clearance. Certain medications have specific administration guidelines, such as administering them with food or on an empty stomach. Consulting drug references and adhering to institutional protocols is imperative for ensuring safe and effective medication practices.

In complex cases, dose calculations may involve multiple steps. For instance, calculating the rate of intravenous infusion of a weight-based medication requires determining the total daily dose, the desired infusion rate (e.g., mg/kg/hour), and then converting that to milliliters per hour based on the drug concentration. These multi-step calculations demand meticulous attention to detail and a thorough understanding of the underlying principles.

Recognizing the potential for errors, especially with complex calculations or high-alert medications, emphasizing the importance of independent double-checking by another qualified healthcare professional is crucial. This practice provides an additional layer of safety, reducing the likelihood of errors reaching the patient. Furthermore, incorporating technology like automated dispensing systems and electronic health records can enhance accuracy and streamline the medication administration process.

Effective communication and documentation are also integral to safe weight-based dosing. Clearly document the child's weight, the calculated dose, the drug administered, the route of administration, and the time of administration. Open communication between healthcare providers, pharmacists, and caregivers is essential for ensuring accurate information transfer and preventing medication errors. Empowering caregivers with clear instructions and answering their questions promotes adherence and safe medication practices at home.

Weight-based dosing is not merely a mathematical exercise, it's a critical patient safety practice. By understanding the principles, performing accurate calculations, considering patient-specific factors, and promoting a culture of safety, healthcare professionals can ensure that children receive the right medication at the right dose, maximizing therapeutic benefits while minimizing the risk of harm. This meticulous approach is fundamental to providing optimal pediatric care.

5.2 Body Surface Area

Body surface area (BSA) provides a more accurate basis for dosing certain medications, especially those with narrow therapeutic indices or those that exhibit significant toxicity. While weight-based dosing is common in pediatrics, BSA offers a better reflection of physiological processes related to drug distribution and elimination. Understanding how to calculate and apply BSA is therefore crucial for safe and effective pediatric pharmacotherapy. This chapter will delve into the practical aspects of BSA calculations and their application in pediatric dosing.

The most commonly used formula for calculating BSA is the Mosteller formula. This formula uses both height and weight to derive a more precise BSA value. It is represented as: BSA (m^2) = (height (cm) x weight (kg) / 3600). Let's dissect this formula. The height in centimeters is multiplied by the weight in kilograms, and this product is then divided by 3600. Finally, the square root of the resulting quotient yields the BSA in square meters. This relatively simple formula provides a readily accessible means to determine BSA in clinical practice.

Consider a practical example. A child measures 90 cm in height and weighs 15 kg. Applying the Mosteller formula: BSA = (90 x 15 / 3600). This simplifies to (1350/3600), then 0.375, which equals approximately 0.61 m^2. This BSA value can then be used to calculate the appropriate dose of a medication prescribed based on BSA.

Another commonly used method for BSA determination is the use of a nomogram. A nomogram is a graphical tool that allows for quick estimation of BSA without performing the actual calculation. It typically consists of three scales: height, weight, and BSA. By drawing a straight line connecting the child's height and weight on their respective scales, the line intersects the BSA scale, indicating the child's BSA. While nomograms offer a convenient alternative, they are less precise than the Mosteller formula.

The application of BSA extends to various clinical scenarios. For instance, chemotherapy dosing often relies on BSA due to the potent nature of these drugs and their potential for serious adverse effects. Accurate dosing based on BSA helps maximize therapeutic efficacy while minimizing the risk of toxicity. Similarly, certain antibiotics and other medications with narrow therapeutic windows are dosed according to BSA to ensure optimal serum concentrations.

Using BSA in dosage calculations involves a straightforward process. Once the BSA is determined using either the Mosteller formula or a nomogram, the prescribed dose per square meter is multiplied by the calculated BSA to obtain the individualized dose for the child. For example, if a medication is prescribed at 50 mg/m^2 and the child's BSA is 0.61 m^2, the calculated dose would be 50 mg/m^2 x 0.61 m^2 = 30.5 mg. This precise dosing strategy ensures that the child receives the correct amount of medication based on their individual body size.

Beyond chemotherapy and antibiotics, several other drug classes benefit from BSA-based dosing. These include certain immunosuppressants used in transplantation, anticonvulsants for managing seizures, and some cardiovascular medications. In these cases, BSA offers a more accurate reflection of the physiological parameters influencing drug distribution and elimination than weight alone. Therefore, BSA-based dosing helps to optimize therapeutic outcomes and minimize the risk of adverse drug reactions.

It's important to remember that BSA is only one factor to consider when determining pediatric drug dosages. Other crucial factors include the child's age, organ function, and the specific pharmacokinetic properties of the medication. Furthermore, close clinical monitoring is essential to assess drug effectiveness and identify any potential adverse effects. By considering these factors in conjunction with BSA, healthcare professionals can make informed decisions about drug therapy and ensure optimal patient care.

While BSA provides a valuable tool for pediatric dosing, it's crucial to acknowledge its limitations. The Mosteller formula, while widely accepted, is based on data from a limited population and may not accurately reflect the BSA of all children. Furthermore, variations in body composition, particularly in obese or malnourished children, can influence drug distribution and clearance, potentially affecting the accuracy of BSA-based dosing.

In conclusion, understanding and applying the concept of body surface area is essential for accurate and safe pediatric drug dosing. The Mosteller formula and nomograms provide practical methods for determining BSA, which is a crucial parameter for calculating individualized drug doses, especially for medications with narrow therapeutic indices or increased toxicity risks. While BSA is a valuable tool, it should be used in conjunction with other clinical considerations and careful monitoring to ensure optimal therapeutic outcomes for pediatric patients. Never solely rely on BSA.

5.3 Age-Based Calculations

While less common than weight-based or body surface area calculations, age can sometimes serve as a starting point for estimating pediatric dosages, especially in emergency situations or when other data is unavailable. It's crucial to understand that age-based calculations are inherently less precise due to the wide variability in children's size and maturity at any given age. They should therefore be used cautiously and replaced with more accurate methods as soon as possible. The primary advantage of age-based methods lies in their simplicity and speed, making them potentially useful in time-sensitive situations.

Several formulas exist for age-based dosing, each with its own limitations and applicability. Fried's rule, for instance, estimates dosage for infants under two years old using the formula (age in months/150) x adult dose. While simple, Fried's rule has fallen out of favor due to its inaccuracy and potential for underdosing, particularly in infants older than six months. Young's rule, designed for children aged 2-12 years, calculates the dose as (age in years/(age in years + 12)) x adult dose. This rule offers slightly better accuracy than Fried's but still suffers from the same inherent limitations of age-based estimations. Beyond 12 years of age, adult dosing is generally considered appropriate, with adjustments made based on individual patient factors.

It's important to emphasize that these rules are estimations, not precise calculations. The actual effective and safe dose for a child can vary significantly based on factors like genetics, organ function, and concurrent medications. Never rely solely on age. Whenever possible, obtain the child's weight and calculate the dose using milligrams per kilogram (mg/kg) or body surface area (BSA) methods, which provide a much more tailored approach. Age-based estimations should be viewed as a temporary measure, used only when absolutely necessary and followed by reassessment and adjustment once more complete information is available.

The limitations of age-based calculations become particularly apparent when considering the wide range of physiological development within any given age group. For example, two children of the same chronological age might have vastly different body weights, impacting drug distribution and clearance. Similarly, variations in organ maturity, particularly liver and kidney function, can significantly influence drug metabolism and excretion. These physiological differences can lead to substantial variability in drug response, even within a narrow age range. Using age alone fails to account for these crucial individual variations.

Further complicating the use of age-based methods is the difference in drug responses between children and adults. Children's developing organ systems often handle drugs differently than mature adult systems. For instance, infants may have reduced drug clearance due to immature kidneys, while adolescents might experience accelerated drug metabolism due to hormonal changes. These developmental factors necessitate careful dose adjustments, which age-based rules alone cannot provide.

In addition to physiological considerations, practical challenges can arise when relying on age. Obtaining an accurate age, particularly in emergency situations, can be difficult. Parental recall might be unreliable, and documentation may not be readily available. In such cases, using age as the sole basis for dosing becomes even more risky. The potential for error in both age determination and subsequent calculation introduces another layer of uncertainty, further emphasizing the need for caution.

To mitigate the risks associated with age-based calculations, always consult a reliable drug reference specific to pediatric patients. These references often provide more detailed guidance on appropriate dosing ranges based on age, weight, and specific clinical indications. They may also include warnings about drug-specific considerations for children, such as altered pharmacokinetics or increased risk of adverse effects. Using these resources in conjunction with clinical judgment can help minimize the potential for medication errors.

When age-based estimations are used, close monitoring of the patient's response to the medication is paramount. Observe for both therapeutic effects and any signs of adverse reactions. If the desired therapeutic effect is not achieved or if toxicity is suspected, reassess the dosage and consider alternative methods for calculation. Continuously evaluate the patient's clinical status and adjust the treatment plan accordingly. This ongoing monitoring is essential for ensuring patient safety when using less precise dosing methods.

Ultimately, the goal in pediatric pharmacotherapy is to achieve optimal therapeutic outcomes while minimizing the risk of harm. While age can sometimes provide a crude estimate of dosage in limited circumstances, striving for more precise and individualized approaches is always preferable. Prioritize weight-based or BSA calculations whenever possible, and reserve age-based methods only for situations where absolutely necessary, always exercising caution and vigilant monitoring. Remember, accurate dosing is fundamental to safe and effective pediatric drug therapy.

5.4 Drug Considerations

Children represent a uniquely vulnerable population when it comes to medication administration. Their developing physiology necessitates careful consideration of drug selection, dosage, and potential adverse effects. This chapter delves into the specific drug-related factors that must be considered when prescribing and administering medications to pediatric patients. We will explore how age-related changes in organ function and body composition influence drug pharmacokinetics, impacting absorption, distribution, metabolism, and excretion. This understanding forms the basis for safe and effective pediatric pharmacotherapy. One crucial aspect of pediatric drug considerations is the immature nature of drug-metabolizing enzymes, particularly in neonates and infants. The liver, the primary site of drug metabolism, is not fully developed at birth. Consequently, many drugs are metabolized more slowly in young children compared to adults. This slower metabolism can lead to increased drug levels and prolonged drug effects, increasing the risk of toxicity. For example, drugs metabolized by the cytochrome P450 enzyme system may require significant dosage adjustments in infants and young children. Clinicians must be aware of these developmental differences and adjust dosages accordingly to avoid adverse events. Monitoring serum drug levels can be particularly valuable in these situations.

Another critical factor is the difference in body composition between children and adults. Children have a higher proportion of total body water and a lower proportion of body fat compared to adults. These differences influence the distribution of drugs within the body. Water-soluble drugs, such as aminoglycosides, may have a larger volume of distribution in children, requiring higher doses to achieve therapeutic concentrations. Conversely, lipid-soluble drugs may have a smaller volume of distribution in young children due to the lower proportion of body fat. Understanding these age-related variations in body composition is essential for accurate dosage calculations.

Furthermore, the blood-brain barrier, which protects the central nervous system from potentially harmful substances, is not fully developed in infants. This increased permeability allows certain drugs to penetrate the brain more readily, potentially leading to enhanced central nervous system effects or toxicity. Therefore, careful consideration must be given to the potential for central nervous system side effects when prescribing medications to infants. Drugs with known central nervous system effects should be used cautiously, with close monitoring for any adverse reactions.

Developmental changes in renal function also significantly impact drug elimination in children. Glomerular filtration rate, a measure of kidney function, is lower in neonates and gradually increases with age, reaching adult levels by late infancy or early childhood. Drugs primarily eliminated by the kidneys, such as many antibiotics, require careful dosage adjustments in younger children to avoid accumulation and toxicity. Monitoring renal function through serum creatinine and urine output is essential for safe and effective drug therapy in this population.

Beyond these physiological considerations, practical aspects of drug administration must also be addressed. Children's preferences for certain dosage forms, such as liquids or chewable tablets, should be considered to ensure medication adherence. The palatability of oral medications can significantly influence a child's willingness to take them. Flavoring agents can often improve the acceptability of liquid medications. Additionally, the availability of age-appropriate formulations and devices, such as calibrated droppers and oral syringes, can enhance the accuracy and safety of drug administration. Educating parents and caregivers about proper medication administration techniques is paramount to ensuring safe and effective treatment.

Moreover, potential drug interactions are a critical concern in pediatric patients, particularly those with chronic medical conditions requiring multiple medications. Polypharmacy, the use of multiple medications concurrently, increases the risk of drug interactions, which can alter drug efficacy or lead to adverse events. Clinicians should carefully review a child's medication list for potential interactions and adjust dosages or medications as needed. Consulting drug interaction databases and resources can provide valuable information for managing polypharmacy in children.

Finally, ongoing monitoring of drug therapy is essential in pediatric patients. Regular assessment of the child's response to medication, including both therapeutic effects and adverse events, is crucial for optimizing treatment. Therapeutic drug monitoring, which involves measuring drug concentrations in blood or other bodily fluids, can be valuable for certain medications with narrow therapeutic indices. This information helps guide dosage adjustments and ensures that drug levels remain within the therapeutic range, maximizing efficacy and minimizing the risk of toxicity. Communication with parents or caregivers about any observed changes in the child's condition is also essential for timely intervention and management of potential adverse events.

5.5 Safety in Pediatrics

Administering medications to children demands a heightened awareness of safety due to their unique physiological vulnerabilities. This chapter delves into critical safety considerations for pediatric dosage calculations, building upon the principles of weight-based dosing, body surface area calculations, and age-based estimations discussed previously. Understanding these nuances is paramount for minimizing medication errors and ensuring optimal therapeutic outcomes in young patients.

One crucial aspect of pediatric medication safety revolves around meticulous verification. Double-checking calculations with a colleague, particularly for high-alert medications like insulin, chemotherapy drugs, and electrolyte solutions, can significantly reduce the risk of errors. Independent verification offers an extra layer of security, ensuring that the calculated dose aligns with established guidelines and the patient's specific needs. Remember, accuracy is non-negotiable when dealing with vulnerable pediatric patients.

Beyond calculations, understanding the specific drug's properties is essential. Consulting comprehensive drug information resources, like the package insert or reputable online databases, is vital. Pay close attention to warnings, contraindications, and adverse effects specific to pediatric populations. For instance, some medications may be contraindicated in neonates due to immature organ function, while others might require dose adjustments based on renal or hepatic function.

Clear communication with the care team is another cornerstone of safe medication practice. This includes effective communication with physicians, nurses, pharmacists, and especially parents or guardians. Providing clear instructions on medication administration, including dose, route, frequency, and potential side effects, empowers caregivers to actively participate in the child's treatment. This collaborative approach strengthens the safety net around the patient.

Precise measurement and administration techniques are equally important. Using calibrated oral syringes or droppers ensures accurate dosing for liquid medications, minimizing the risk of overdosing or underdosing. Crushing tablets or opening capsules should only be done when absolutely necessary and after verifying that the medication is suitable for such manipulation. Some medications have enteric coatings or sustained-release formulations that should never be compromised.

Monitoring for adverse drug reactions is a continuous process in pediatric care. Children may exhibit different or more pronounced adverse effects compared to adults. Being vigilant for any unusual signs or symptoms, and promptly reporting them to the physician, is crucial for early intervention and mitigating potential harm. This proactive approach underscores the importance of close observation in pediatric pharmacotherapy.

Effective documentation forms an integral part of safe medication administration. Recording the calculated dose, the medication administered, the time of administration, and the route used provides a clear audit trail. This meticulous documentation facilitates communication among healthcare providers, enhances continuity of care, and serves as a valuable resource for evaluating the effectiveness and safety of the prescribed therapy.

Patient education is a vital component of medication safety, especially in pediatrics. Explain the medication's purpose, dosage, and potential side effects to parents or guardians in a clear and understandable manner. Addressing their concerns and emphasizing the importance of adherence to the prescribed regimen promotes patient safety and optimizes treatment outcomes. Empowered caregivers are better equipped to manage their child's medications safely and effectively.

Understanding pharmacokinetic principles specific to children is crucial for safe medication practice. Children have different rates of drug absorption, distribution, metabolism, and excretion compared to adults. For example, their immature liver function may necessitate dose reductions for medications that are primarily metabolized by the liver. Similarly, differences in body composition can influence drug distribution, impacting the effective dose at the target site.

Drug interactions pose a significant risk in pediatric patients, particularly those receiving multiple medications. Polypharmacy, or the concurrent use of multiple drugs, increases the potential for drug-drug interactions. Being aware of potential interactions and adjusting dosages accordingly is crucial. Consulting drug interaction databases or seeking guidance from a pharmacist can help mitigate these risks and ensure safe medication management.

Age-related physiological changes further influence drug disposition in children. Neonates, for instance, have underdeveloped renal function, requiring careful dose adjustments for drugs primarily eliminated by the kidneys. As children grow and develop, their organ function matures, necessitating age-appropriate dose adjustments. This dynamic nature of pediatric pharmacokinetics underscores the need for ongoing assessment and dose individualization.

Finally, fostering a culture of safety within the healthcare setting is paramount. This includes promoting error reporting systems that encourage open communication and facilitate learning from mistakes. Regular training and education on pediatric medication safety principles, including dosage calculations, drug interactions, and adverse event monitoring, empower healthcare professionals to provide optimal care and minimize medication-related risks. Creating a safe and supportive environment benefits both patients and practitioners.

6 Geriatric Dosage Considerations

As individuals age, physiological changes occur that significantly impact how medications are processed within the body. These age-related alterations necessitate careful consideration when determining appropriate drug dosages for older adults. Ignoring these changes can lead to adverse drug reactions and diminished therapeutic efficacy. Therefore, understanding the pharmacokinetic changes associated with aging is crucial for safe and effective medication management in this population.

One key change is the decrease in glomerular filtration rate (GFR), a measure of kidney function. This decline often begins in the fourth decade of life and continues progressively. As GFR decreases, the kidneys become less efficient at clearing drugs from the body, potentially leading to drug accumulation and toxicity. Drugs primarily eliminated by renal excretion require careful dosage adjustments based on the patient's estimated GFR. Creatinine clearance, readily obtained from serum creatinine levels and patient demographics, provides a practical estimate of GFR for dosage adjustments.

Absorption of medications can also be affected by aging. While the overall extent of absorption may not be significantly altered for many drugs, the rate of absorption can slow down. This is due to factors such as decreased gastric motility and reduced splanchnic blood flow. Delayed absorption can prolong the time to reach peak drug concentrations, but it generally doesn't affect the overall amount of drug absorbed. However, for drugs with a narrow therapeutic index, even minor changes in absorption rate can have clinical implications.

Distribution of drugs within the body is also impacted by age-related changes in body composition. Older adults typically have a lower proportion of lean body mass and a higher proportion of body fat. For lipophilic drugs, this means a larger volume of distribution, which can lead to a longer elimination half-life and prolonged drug effects. Conversely, hydrophilic drugs may have a smaller volume of distribution, potentially leading to higher initial drug concentrations. These changes necessitate careful monitoring and potential dosage adjustments to ensure therapeutic efficacy and minimize adverse effects.

Hepatic metabolism, the process by which the liver breaks down drugs, also declines with age. This reduction in metabolic capacity can be attributed to decreased liver mass, reduced hepatic blood flow, and diminished activity of drug-metabolizing enzymes. The impact of these changes varies considerably among individuals and across different drug classes. For drugs extensively metabolized by the liver, reduced clearance can lead to elevated drug levels and an increased risk of toxicity. Consequently, starting with lower doses and titrating slowly based on patient response is often recommended.

The risk of drug interactions increases substantially in older adults due to polypharmacy, the concurrent use of multiple medications. This is common in this population due to the higher prevalence of chronic conditions requiring pharmacotherapy. Drug interactions can occur when two or more drugs compete for the same metabolic pathway or binding sites, or when one drug alters the absorption, distribution, metabolism, or excretion of another. These interactions can either enhance or diminish the effects of the involved drugs, potentially leading to adverse reactions or therapeutic failure. A thorough medication review, including over-the-counter medications and herbal supplements, is essential to identify and minimize potential drug interactions.

Understanding age-related changes in drug absorption, distribution, metabolism, and excretion is foundational for safe and effective medication management in the geriatric population. These changes necessitate careful consideration of patient-specific factors, including renal and hepatic function, body composition, and concurrent medications. By acknowledging these physiological alterations and implementing appropriate dosage adjustments, healthcare professionals can optimize therapeutic outcomes and minimize the risk of adverse drug reactions in older adults. This individualized approach is crucial for ensuring the safe and effective use of medications in this vulnerable population. Regularly reviewing medications and monitoring patient response are essential components of providing optimal geriatric care. Additionally, educating patients and their families about the importance of medication adherence and potential adverse effects empowers them to actively participate in their care and enhances medication safety. Furthermore, collaborating with pharmacists and other healthcare professionals can provide additional expertise in managing complex medication regimens and minimizing the risk of drug-related problems in older adults. Ultimately, a comprehensive and collaborative approach is essential for ensuring the safe and effective use of medications in this population, promoting optimal health outcomes and improving their quality of life.

6.1 Pharmacokinetic Changes

Aging brings about a cascade of physiological changes that significantly impact how the body processes medications. These age-related alterations necessitate careful consideration of drug dosages to ensure therapeutic efficacy and minimize the risk of adverse effects in older adults. This chapter will delve into the specific pharmacokinetic changes that occur with aging and how they influence drug disposition.

Absorption, the initial step in drug action, can be altered in older adults due to several factors. Decreased gastric acid production, a common occurrence with age, can affect the dissolution and absorption of certain medications, particularly those that require an acidic environment for optimal absorption. Furthermore, reduced intestinal blood flow can slow down the rate at which drugs are absorbed into the systemic circulation. Changes in gastrointestinal motility, such as delayed gastric emptying, can also influence drug absorption patterns, leading to unpredictable drug levels. These age-related changes in absorption, while not always clinically significant for all drugs, can contribute to variability in drug response.

Once absorbed, a drug's distribution throughout the body is also influenced by age-related physiological shifts. A decrease in total body water, coupled with an increase in body fat percentage, is commonly observed in older adults. These changes can alter the volume of distribution for certain medications, leading to higher plasma concentrations of water-soluble drugs and prolonged half-lives for fat-soluble drugs. Additionally, a decline in serum albumin levels, a protein responsible for binding many drugs in the bloodstream, can increase the fraction of unbound (free) drug, potentially leading to increased drug activity and a higher risk of toxicity. It's crucial to consider these changes when interpreting drug levels and adjusting dosages.

Metabolism, the process by which the body breaks down drugs, is primarily carried out by the liver. With age, hepatic blood flow and liver mass often decrease, leading to a reduction in the metabolic capacity of the liver. This decline in liver function can result in slower drug metabolism, leading to increased drug exposure and a heightened risk of adverse effects, especially for drugs with a narrow therapeutic index. Careful monitoring of drug levels and appropriate dosage adjustments are essential for ensuring safe and effective drug therapy in older adults. Consideration should also be given to potential drug-drug interactions, which are more likely to occur in older adults due to polypharmacy (the use of multiple medications).

The final stage of pharmacokinetics is excretion, primarily handled by the kidneys. Age-related decline in renal function, as measured by glomerular filtration rate (GFR), is a common finding in older individuals. This reduced kidney function can significantly impact the elimination of drugs that are primarily excreted renally, leading to drug accumulation and an increased risk of toxicity. Accurate assessment of renal function using creatinine clearance or estimated GFR is crucial for determining appropriate drug dosages in older adults. Adjustments in dosage regimens, based on individual renal function, are often necessary to avoid drug accumulation and adverse effects.

Understanding these age-related pharmacokinetic changes is paramount for healthcare professionals involved in the care of older adults. It underscores the importance of individualized drug therapy based on a patient's specific physiological characteristics and comorbidities. Regular monitoring of drug levels and vigilant assessment for potential drug-related adverse events are crucial components of safe and effective medication management in this population. By considering the complex interplay of these factors, healthcare providers can optimize drug therapy and improve outcomes for older adults. Remember, the goal is to achieve therapeutic drug concentrations while minimizing the risk of adverse effects. This requires a nuanced approach that acknowledges the dynamic interplay of age, physiology, and pharmacology.

6.2 Drug Interactions

Polypharmacy, the concurrent use of multiple medications, is a common occurrence in older adults. This practice significantly increases the risk of drug interactions, a crucial consideration in geriatric pharmacotherapy. Drug interactions occur when the effects of one drug are altered by the presence of another drug, food, or other substance. These interactions can lead to a variety of consequences, ranging from reduced therapeutic efficacy to enhanced adverse effects, impacting patient outcomes and healthcare costs. Understanding the mechanisms and potential consequences of these interactions is paramount for safe and effective medication management in the elderly.

One major mechanism of drug interaction is altered absorption. For example, antacids, frequently used by older adults for heartburn, can interfere with the absorption of certain antibiotics, such as tetracycline, by forming insoluble complexes. This reduces the antibiotic's bioavailability and potentially compromises treatment. Conversely, drugs that increase gastric emptying, like metoclopramide, may enhance the absorption of rapidly dissolving medications. It's important to consider the timing of medication administration to minimize such interactions.

Drug distribution, the process by which a drug is transported throughout the body, can also be affected by other medications. Competition for protein binding sites in the bloodstream is a common mechanism. Many drugs bind to plasma proteins, like albumin. When two drugs compete for the same binding site, the drug with less affinity can be displaced, resulting in an increased free fraction of that drug. This can lead to elevated drug concentrations and a heightened risk of adverse effects. Warfarin, a commonly prescribed anticoagulant, is highly protein-bound and susceptible to displacement by other drugs. Close monitoring of the international normalized ratio (INR), a measure of blood clotting time, is crucial when introducing new medications to patients on warfarin.

Metabolism, the process by which the body chemically modifies drugs, is another critical area for potential interactions. The liver plays a central role in drug metabolism, primarily through cytochrome P450 enzymes. Some drugs, known as enzyme inhibitors, can reduce the activity of these enzymes, leading to decreased metabolism and accumulation of other drugs metabolized by the same pathway. Grapefruit juice, for instance, inhibits CYP3A4, an enzyme involved in the metabolism of numerous drugs, including statins and some calcium channel blockers. This can result in increased drug levels and greater risk of side effects. Conversely, enzyme inducers can accelerate drug metabolism, reducing drug effectiveness. Smoking, for example, induces CYP1A2, which metabolizes drugs like clozapine, an antipsychotic medication.

Excretion, the process of removing drugs and their metabolites from the body, is primarily carried out by the kidneys. Drug interactions can occur when drugs alter renal blood flow or compete for the same transport mechanisms involved in renal excretion. Nonsteroidal anti-inflammatory drugs (NSAIDs) can reduce renal blood flow, potentially impacting the excretion of other drugs, including lithium and digoxin. This can lead to increased serum concentrations and toxicity. Monitoring renal function, particularly in older adults, is vital when managing multiple medications.

Beyond these pharmacokinetic interactions, pharmacodynamic interactions can also occur. These involve the combined effects of drugs acting on the same physiological system or receptor. For example, the concurrent use of two antihypertensive medications, such as a beta-blocker and a calcium channel blocker, can lead to additive effects and excessive blood pressure lowering. While sometimes intentional for therapeutic benefit, this can also result in orthostatic hypotension, an abrupt drop in blood pressure upon standing, increasing the risk of falls, a significant concern in the elderly. Similarly, combining medications that have sedative effects, such as benzodiazepines and opioids, can lead to profound sedation and respiratory depression.

In managing polypharmacy in geriatric patients, meticulous medication reconciliation is essential. A thorough review of all prescribed and over-the-counter medications, including herbal supplements, should be conducted at each patient visit. Potential drug interactions should be identified and assessed for clinical significance. Therapeutic drug monitoring, where applicable, can help optimize drug levels and minimize the risk of toxicity. Patient education is crucial. Empowering patients with knowledge about their medications and potential interactions can enhance adherence and improve outcomes. Open communication with patients and caregivers encourages reporting of any unusual symptoms that may indicate a drug interaction. Finally, a collaborative approach involving physicians, pharmacists, and other healthcare professionals is essential for managing polypharmacy effectively and minimizing the risk of drug interactions in older adults.

7 Clinical Applications & Case Studies

Let's delve into the complexities of dosage adjustments in specific patient populations, focusing on renal impairment, hepatic dysfunction, critical care scenarios, oncology calculations, and pain management. These areas demand careful consideration due to altered drug pharmacokinetics and pharmacodynamics.

Renal impairment significantly impacts drug clearance. A diminished glomerular filtration rate (GFR) necessitates dosage reductions for drugs primarily excreted by the kidneys. Creatinine clearance, often estimated using the Cockcroft-Gault equation, serves as a valuable tool for assessing renal function and guiding dosage adjustments. For example, a patient with a GFR of 30 mL/min may require a significantly lower dose of a renally cleared antibiotic compared to a patient with normal renal function. Ignoring this could lead to drug accumulation and toxicity. We'll examine specific examples of drug adjustments based on varying degrees of renal impairment.

Hepatic dysfunction presents another challenge. The liver plays a crucial role in drug metabolism. In patients with liver disease, drug metabolism may be compromised, leading to elevated drug levels and increased risk of adverse effects. Unlike renal function, liver function is harder to quantify, making dosage adjustments less precise. Child-Pugh and MELD scores provide some guidance, but clinical judgment and close monitoring are essential. We will discuss how the pharmacokinetic parameters of specific drugs are altered in hepatic impairment and the strategies for mitigating risks.

The critical care setting presents unique challenges. Critically ill patients often experience dramatic physiological changes that affect drug disposition. These include alterations in volume of distribution, protein binding, and organ perfusion. Furthermore, therapeutic drug monitoring becomes crucial in this context to ensure optimal drug levels are achieved. We'll explore how these factors impact drug dosing in commonly encountered critical care scenarios, such as sepsis and acute respiratory distress syndrome.

Oncology calculations require a different approach. Chemotherapy dosing often involves calculating body surface area (BSA), especially in pediatric oncology. This approach accounts for variations in body size and composition. Furthermore, chemotherapy regimens often involve complex dosing schedules and combination therapies, adding another layer of complexity. We'll delve into the intricacies of calculating BSA and navigating the nuances of various chemotherapeutic protocols.

Pain management presents its own set of dosage dilemmas. Chronic pain conditions often necessitate long-term opioid therapy, which requires careful titration to balance pain relief with the risk of adverse effects. Patient-controlled analgesia (PCA) provides a degree of autonomy for patients to manage their pain, but requires careful programming to ensure safety. We will explore the principles of opioid dosing, including equianalgesic conversions and the importance of individualized therapy. Furthermore, we will consider the role of adjuvant analgesics in enhancing pain control and reducing opioid requirements.

Consider a case involving a 75-year-old woman with chronic kidney disease requiring antibiotic therapy. Her estimated creatinine clearance indicates moderate renal impairment. Selecting an appropriate antibiotic and adjusting the dosage based on her renal function is crucial to prevent drug accumulation and potential toxicity. This scenario highlights the importance of integrating knowledge of pharmacokinetics, renal function assessment, and drug-specific considerations.

Another case might involve a patient with cirrhosis receiving a medication metabolized by the liver. Close monitoring for signs of drug toxicity is necessary, and dosage adjustments may be required. This illustrates the challenges posed by hepatic dysfunction and the importance of clinical judgment.

In a critical care setting, consider a patient with septic shock receiving a vasopressor. Titrating the dose to achieve the desired hemodynamic effect while minimizing adverse effects requires careful monitoring and frequent dosage adjustments based on the patient's response. This emphasizes the dynamic nature of critical care and the need for continuous assessment and intervention.

An oncology patient receiving chemotherapy may require dosage adjustments based on their BSA. Accurate calculation of BSA and careful adherence to the prescribed protocol are crucial for maximizing efficacy and minimizing toxicity. This demonstrates the specialized calculations necessary in oncology and the importance of precision.

Finally, a patient with chronic pain requiring opioid therapy presents a complex challenge. Careful titration based on pain response and side effects, along with consideration of adjuvant therapies, is essential for optimizing pain management. This underscores the importance of individualized therapy and the complexities of long-term pain management. These case studies demonstrate the practical application of the principles discussed in this chapter, bridging the gap between theory and clinical practice.

7.1 Renal Impairment

Kidney function is paramount when determining appropriate drug dosages. Compromised renal function can significantly alter drug clearance, leading to accumulation and potential toxicity. This chapter will equip you with the knowledge and skills to safely and effectively adjust drug doses for patients with varying degrees of renal impairment. Understanding the impact of renal function on drug disposition is essential for any healthcare professional involved in medication management.

The kidneys play a vital role in eliminating drugs from the body. When renal function declines, the ability to clear drugs diminishes, necessitating dosage adjustments. The severity of renal impairment is often quantified by estimating the glomerular filtration rate (GFR). GFR, typically reported in milliliters per minute, represents the volume of plasma filtered by the kidneys per unit of time. Several equations exist for estimating GFR, including the Cockcroft-Gault and Modification of Diet in Renal Disease (MDRD) formulas, each with its own advantages and limitations. Choosing the appropriate equation depends on factors like patient demographics and clinical context. Accurate GFR estimation is the cornerstone of appropriate dose adjustment in renal impairment.

Once GFR is estimated, it's crucial to consult reputable resources like drug package inserts or clinical pharmacology references. These resources often provide specific recommendations for dose adjustments based on GFR categories, typically ranging from normal function to end-stage renal disease. Recommendations might include reducing the dose, extending the dosing interval, or both. However, a "one-size-fits-all" approach doesn't exist. Individualized dosing is key, taking into account not only GFR but also patient-specific factors such as age, weight, comorbidities, and concomitant medications. Therapeutic drug monitoring, where applicable, can further refine dosing decisions by measuring drug levels and ensuring they remain within the therapeutic range.

Beyond GFR, understanding the drug's pharmacokinetic properties is crucial for optimal dose adjustment. Consider the drug's route of elimination. If renal excretion is the primary route, dosage adjustments are more critical. For drugs with significant non-renal elimination pathways (e.g., hepatic metabolism or biliary excretion), the impact of renal impairment may be less pronounced. The drug's therapeutic index, the ratio between the effective and toxic dose, also informs decision-making. Drugs with a narrow therapeutic index require more careful monitoring and smaller dose adjustments to avoid toxicity. Knowledge of these pharmacokinetic principles allows for more nuanced and individualized dosing strategies.

Consider the case of a patient with moderate renal impairment (GFR 30-59 mL/min) prescribed an antibiotic primarily eliminated by the kidneys. Referring to the drug's package insert reveals a recommended dose reduction of 50% for this GFR range. However, the patient is also elderly and frail, potentially increasing their susceptibility to drug toxicity. In this scenario, starting with a lower dose than the standard 50% reduction and closely monitoring for efficacy and adverse effects may be a safer approach. This highlights the importance of integrating clinical judgment with established guidelines.

Another common scenario involves drugs that require dose adjustment based on creatinine clearance, a measure related to GFR. Creatinine clearance can be estimated using the Cockcroft-Gault equation, which incorporates age, weight, and serum creatinine concentration. While less precise than measured creatinine clearance, estimated values are often sufficient for guiding dose adjustments. Accurate creatinine measurements are essential for reliable calculations, and clinicians should be aware of factors that can influence creatinine levels, such as muscle mass and dietary intake.

Drugs with active metabolites that are renally cleared require special attention. Accumulation of these metabolites can contribute to toxicity even if the parent drug is appropriately dosed. Understanding the pharmacokinetic profile of both the parent drug and its metabolites is essential for safe and effective medication management in renal impairment. For instance, morphine is metabolized to active metabolites that are renally excreted. In patients with renal dysfunction, these metabolites can accumulate, leading to prolonged opioid effects and an increased risk of respiratory depression. Therefore, dose adjustments and careful monitoring are crucial when prescribing morphine to patients with impaired renal function.

Always be vigilant for drug-drug interactions, particularly in patients with renal impairment. Drugs that compete for renal excretion pathways can increase the risk of toxicity. For example, co-administration of two drugs that are both primarily eliminated by the kidneys can lead to decreased clearance of one or both drugs, potentially resulting in adverse effects. Careful review of a patient's medication list is essential to identify and manage potential drug-drug interactions. Consulting drug interaction databases and pharmacology resources can help assess the risk and guide appropriate interventions. Open communication with the patient's healthcare team, including pharmacists and other specialists, is vital for optimizing medication regimens in patients with complex medical conditions and polypharmacy.

This iterative process, involving GFR assessment, consultation of reliable resources, consideration of pharmacokinetic principles, and careful monitoring, empowers clinicians to navigate the complexities of drug dosing in renal impairment. By integrating these principles into practice, healthcare professionals can optimize medication therapy, minimize adverse effects, and improve patient outcomes. This dedication to personalized, informed prescribing is fundamental to ensuring patient safety and therapeutic efficacy. Remember that ongoing assessment and reassessment are crucial in dynamic clinical settings.

7.2 Hepatic Dysfunction

The liver, a central processing hub for medications, plays a crucial role in drug metabolism. When liver function is compromised, the ability to process drugs effectively diminishes, leading to potential drug accumulation and toxicity. This necessitates careful dosage adjustments to maintain therapeutic efficacy while minimizing the risk of adverse events. Understanding the impact of hepatic dysfunction on drug pharmacokinetics is essential for safe and effective pharmacotherapy.

Liver disease encompasses a wide spectrum of conditions, ranging from mild fatty liver to severe cirrhosis and acute liver failure. The severity of the dysfunction directly correlates with the degree of impairment in drug metabolism. Mild dysfunction may only require minor dosage adjustments, while severe impairment often necessitates significant reductions or even avoidance of certain medications altogether. Assessment of liver function is therefore a critical first step in determining appropriate drug dosing for patients with hepatic impairment.

Several methods exist to assess liver function, each offering unique insights. Commonly used tests include serum albumin, bilirubin, prothrombin time (PT), and the international normalized ratio (INR). These markers provide information about the liver's synthetic and metabolic capacity. More specific tests, such as the Child-Pugh score and the Model for End-Stage Liver Disease (MELD) score, provide a more comprehensive assessment of liver function and are often used to guide dosage adjustments for drugs with a narrow therapeutic index.

Drugs are primarily metabolized through two main phases: Phase I and Phase II. Phase I reactions typically involve oxidation, reduction, or hydrolysis, while Phase II reactions involve conjugation with various molecules, making the drug more water-soluble for excretion. Hepatic dysfunction can affect both phases, but the impact can vary depending on the specific drug and the nature of the impairment. For example, cirrhosis can significantly reduce the activity of cytochrome P450 enzymes, which are essential for many Phase I reactions. This can lead to reduced clearance and increased plasma concentrations of drugs primarily metabolized by these enzymes.

Dosage adjustments in patients with hepatic dysfunction must be individualized based on the severity of the impairment, the specific drug being used, and the patient's overall clinical status. General guidelines exist for many drugs, but these should be viewed as starting points and adjusted based on therapeutic drug monitoring and close observation for adverse events. For some drugs, no specific dosage adjustments are recommended, while for others, significant reductions or alternative therapies may be necessary.

Drugs with a high hepatic extraction ratio are particularly susceptible to changes in liver function. These drugs are efficiently removed from the bloodstream by the liver during first-pass metabolism. When liver function is impaired, the extraction ratio decreases, leading to a disproportionately large increase in systemic drug exposure. This can result in significant toxicity if dosages are not adjusted accordingly.

Consulting drug information resources specific to hepatic impairment is crucial for making informed dosing decisions. These resources provide detailed information about the effects of liver disease on drug pharmacokinetics, recommended dosage adjustments, and alternative therapeutic options. Pharmacists play a vital role in interpreting this information and providing individualized recommendations based on each patient's unique circumstances.

Monitoring patients closely for both therapeutic efficacy and adverse effects is essential when adjusting dosages for hepatic dysfunction. Therapeutic drug monitoring, where available, can provide valuable information about drug concentrations and help guide further dosage adjustments. Close communication between healthcare professionals, including physicians, pharmacists, and nurses, is crucial to ensure optimal patient outcomes.

Beyond drug-specific adjustments, supportive care measures can be implemented to optimize liver function and minimize the risk of complications. These measures may include nutritional support, avoidance of hepatotoxic substances, and management of underlying liver disease. Addressing these factors can contribute to improved drug tolerance and overall patient well-being.

Considering the complexities surrounding hepatic dysfunction and its influence on drug metabolism, a systematic approach to dosage adjustment is crucial. This includes careful assessment of liver function, understanding the metabolic pathway of the drug, consulting reliable drug information resources, individualizing dosage regimens, and closely monitoring patients for efficacy and toxicity. By integrating these principles, healthcare professionals can ensure the safe and effective use of medications in patients with compromised liver function, promoting optimal therapeutic outcomes and minimizing the risk of adverse events. This individualized and meticulous approach ensures that even in the face of hepatic challenges, medication therapy remains a tool for healing and improvement, not a source of further complications.

7.3 Critical Care Dosing

The critically ill patient presents unique challenges in drug dosing. Physiological derangements common in these patients significantly alter pharmacokinetics, impacting drug absorption, distribution, metabolism, and excretion. Understanding these alterations is paramount for effective and safe drug therapy. This chapter will explore the intricacies of drug dosing in the critical care setting, focusing on practical application and problem-solving. We will delve into the impact of organ dysfunction, altered volume of distribution, and therapeutic drug monitoring, equipping you with the tools to make informed dosing decisions.

Consider the impact of hypoperfusion, often seen in septic shock. Reduced blood flow to the gut can significantly impair drug absorption, leading to subtherapeutic levels even with standard doses. Conversely, drugs administered intravenously may reach higher-than-expected concentrations due to decreased distribution volume secondary to fluid shifts and capillary leak. This highlights the importance of continuous monitoring and dose adjustments based on patient response. For instance, a patient receiving an aminoglycoside antibiotic might require therapeutic drug monitoring to ensure efficacy while minimizing the risk of nephrotoxicity, a risk exacerbated in the critically ill.

The volume of distribution (Vd) can fluctuate drastically in critical illness. Conditions like sepsis, burns, and acute kidney injury can dramatically alter fluid balance, impacting drug distribution. A drug with a large Vd, such as amiodarone, may require a larger loading dose to achieve therapeutic levels in a patient with an expanded Vd due to fluid overload. This necessitates a thorough assessment of the patient's fluid status and careful calculation of loading and maintenance doses. Failure to account for changes in Vd can lead to either subtherapeutic or toxic drug levels, highlighting the importance of incorporating this parameter into dosing decisions.

Hepatic dysfunction further complicates drug dosing in critical care. The liver plays a crucial role in drug metabolism, and its impairment can lead to accumulation of drugs metabolized by the liver, increasing the risk of adverse effects. Propofol, for example, is heavily reliant on hepatic metabolism. In a patient with liver failure, the dosage of propofol must be significantly reduced to avoid prolonged sedation or even respiratory depression. Close monitoring of patient response and drug levels are vital in such scenarios.

Renal dysfunction also presents significant challenges. Many drugs are renally cleared, and a decline in kidney function can lead to drug accumulation and toxicity. Vancomycin, a commonly used antibiotic in critical care, is primarily excreted by the kidneys. Dosage adjustments based on creatinine clearance are essential to prevent accumulation and potential nephrotoxicity. Furthermore, continuous renal replacement therapy (CRRT) can further alter drug clearance, requiring specific dosing strategies and careful monitoring.

Therapeutic drug monitoring (TDM) becomes an indispensable tool in the critical care setting. For drugs with a narrow therapeutic index, such as digoxin and phenytoin, TDM helps optimize drug efficacy while minimizing the risk of toxicity. By measuring drug concentrations at specific time points, clinicians can individualize dosing regimens and ensure therapeutic levels are maintained. This is particularly crucial in patients with fluctuating organ function, where predicting drug levels based on standard dosing protocols can be unreliable.

In addition to organ dysfunction, critical illness often leads to altered protein binding. Many drugs bind to plasma proteins, and only the unbound fraction is pharmacologically active. Conditions like hypoalbuminemia, common in critically ill patients, can increase the free fraction of highly protein-bound drugs like phenytoin, potentially leading to toxicity. Monitoring free drug levels, rather than total drug levels, provides a more accurate assessment of the active drug concentration and guides appropriate dosage adjustments.

The critically ill patient often requires multiple medications concurrently, increasing the risk of drug interactions. These interactions can alter drug absorption, metabolism, or excretion, leading to unpredictable drug levels and potentially serious adverse events. For example, the co-administration of certain antibiotics with warfarin can potentiate warfarin's anticoagulant effect, increasing the risk of bleeding. A thorough understanding of potential drug interactions is paramount in the critical care setting.

Pharmacokinetic principles are not static concepts in critical care. They dynamically change with the patient's physiological state. Regular reassessment of organ function, fluid status, and drug levels is crucial for safe and effective drug therapy. The ability to interpret these parameters and adjust dosages accordingly is essential for optimizing patient outcomes. Employing a systematic approach, integrating clinical assessment with pharmacokinetic principles, empowers the clinician to navigate the complexities of critical care dosing. Understanding the interplay of these factors enables informed decisions, promoting patient safety and maximizing therapeutic efficacy in this challenging environment. Remember, meticulous attention to detail and continuous monitoring are cornerstones of effective drug therapy in the critically ill.

7.4 Oncology Calculations

Chemotherapy dosing is complex, demanding meticulous calculations that go beyond basic arithmetic. It's a domain where precision isn't just preferred, it's essential for patient safety and treatment efficacy. This chapter equips you with the tools to confidently navigate the intricacies of oncology calculations. We'll dissect crucial formulas and explore practical examples, emphasizing the specific nuances that distinguish oncology dosing.

A cornerstone of chemotherapy dosing is the body surface area (BSA). Why BSA? Because anticancer drugs often exhibit a narrow therapeutic index – the difference between a therapeutic dose and a toxic dose is small. BSA offers a more accurate reflection of the body's overall metabolic capacity and drug distribution compared to weight alone. The most common method for BSA calculation is the Mosteller formula: BSA (m^2) = (Height (cm) x Weight (kg) / 3600). Let's illustrate. A patient is 175 cm tall and weighs 70 kg. Applying the formula: BSA = (175 x 70 / 3600) = 3.40 1.84 m^2. This calculated BSA then becomes a crucial factor in determining the patient's chemotherapy dosage.

Now, consider the Calvert formula, used to calculate the dose of carboplatin, a common chemotherapeutic agent. The formula is: Total Carboplatin Dose (mg) = Target AUC x (GFR + 25). The Target AUC (Area Under the Curve) represents the desired drug exposure, typically determined by the specific cancer being treated. GFR stands for Glomerular Filtration Rate, an indicator of kidney function. Let's say a patient has a Target AUC of 6 and a GFR of 100 ml/min. Their Carboplatin dose would be: 6 x (100 + 25) = 750 mg. This formula highlights the importance of considering organ function in chemotherapy dosing. Impaired kidney function, as indicated by a lower GFR, necessitates a reduced carboplatin dose to prevent toxicity.

Dosage calculations for targeted therapies, a newer class of anticancer drugs, often differ from traditional chemotherapy. These agents typically target specific molecular pathways involved in cancer growth and are often administered as fixed doses, unlike the BSA-based dosing of many conventional chemotherapeutics. For example, a patient might receive a monoclonal antibody at a fixed dose of, say, 150 mg regardless of their BSA. However, even with fixed doses, considerations like frequency and duration of treatment are crucial and dictated by the specific drug regimen.

Another complexity arises with dose adjustments. Chemotherapy often requires dose modifications based on a patient's response to treatment and tolerance of side effects. Myelosuppression, a decrease in bone marrow activity leading to reduced blood cell counts, is a common side effect of chemotherapy. If a patient experiences significant myelosuppression, their subsequent chemotherapy dose may be reduced. This reduction might be expressed as a percentage of the original dose. For example, if a patient's original dose was 800 mg and requires a 25% dose reduction, the adjusted dose would be 800 mg \item (0.25 x 800 mg) = 600 mg.

Furthermore, combination chemotherapy regimens, which involve administering multiple drugs concurrently, introduce another layer of complexity. Each drug within the regimen might have its own specific dosing schedule and calculations. For example, a regimen might involve one drug dosed based on BSA, another administered as a fixed dose, and a third given as a continuous infusion over a specified time period. Accurately calculating and administering each drug within these complex regimens demands careful attention to detail and a thorough understanding of the specific protocol.

Beyond BSA, other patient-specific factors may influence dosage calculations. Age, comorbidities, and concomitant medications can all impact drug clearance and potentially warrant dose adjustments. Geriatric patients, for instance, often experience age-related decline in renal and hepatic function, impacting drug metabolism and elimination. Consequently, lower doses might be necessary to avoid toxicity. Similarly, patients with pre-existing liver or kidney disease may require dose modifications based on their individual organ function.

Finally, it's crucial to recognize that oncology calculations are not a static process. Ongoing monitoring of the patient's response to therapy, including laboratory results and clinical assessment, is essential. This allows for dynamic dose adjustments throughout the treatment course, ensuring both efficacy and safety. Regular evaluation of kidney and liver function, blood cell counts, and other relevant parameters provides the necessary data for informed decision-making regarding dosage adjustments. Remember, in the realm of oncology calculations, meticulousness is paramount. Every step, from initial calculation to subsequent adjustments, demands a focused and precise approach.

7.5 Pain Management

Effective pain management is a cornerstone of patient care, requiring a nuanced understanding of pharmacology, patient-specific factors, and analgesic principles. Calculating appropriate dosages is crucial for achieving optimal pain relief while minimizing adverse effects. This chapter builds upon the foundational concepts of dosage calculations and pharmacokinetics, applying them to the complex landscape of pain medications. We will delve into various analgesic classes, exploring their mechanisms of action and considering the factors that influence their dosage and administration.

Opioid analgesics, including morphine, fentanyl, and oxycodone, are potent pain relievers that act on opioid receptors in the central nervous system. Calculating opioid dosages requires careful consideration of the patient's age, weight, renal function, and hepatic function. Titration, the process of gradually adjusting the dose to achieve optimal pain relief while minimizing side effects, is paramount in opioid therapy. Equianalgesic charts, which provide conversion factors between different opioids, are invaluable tools for switching between medications or routes of administration. However, these charts should be used with caution, recognizing that individual patient responses can vary.

Nonsteroidal anti-inflammatory drugs (NSAIDs) like ibuprofen and naproxen provide analgesia by inhibiting cyclooxygenase enzymes, thereby reducing inflammation and pain. Calculating NSAID dosages typically involves standard adult doses, but adjustments may be necessary for patients with renal impairment or a history of gastrointestinal bleeding. Combining NSAIDs with other analgesics, such as opioids, can provide synergistic pain relief, allowing for lower doses of each medication and potentially reducing side effects.

Acetaminophen, a commonly used analgesic and antipyretic, is effective for mild to moderate pain. Calculating acetaminophen dosages is generally straightforward, but caution must be exercised to avoid exceeding the maximum daily dose, as overdoses can cause severe liver damage. Monitoring liver function tests is crucial, especially in patients with pre-existing liver disease or those taking multiple medications that are metabolized by the liver.

Adjuvant analgesics, such as antidepressants and anticonvulsants, can enhance pain relief when used in conjunction with traditional analgesics. These medications target different pain pathways and can be particularly effective for neuropathic pain, a type of chronic pain caused by nerve damage. Calculating dosages for adjuvant analgesics often requires individualized titration based on patient response and tolerability.

Patient-controlled analgesia (PCA) is a method of pain management that allows patients to self-administer predetermined doses of analgesics, typically opioids, via an intravenous pump. Calculating PCA dosages involves determining the basal infusion rate, the bolus dose, and the lockout interval. Careful monitoring and adjustments are necessary to ensure patient safety and optimize pain control.

Calculating dosages for epidural and intrathecal analgesia, techniques used to deliver analgesics directly to the spinal cord, requires specialized knowledge and meticulous calculations. Factors such as drug concentration, volume, and infusion rate must be carefully considered to ensure accurate delivery and avoid complications.

The management of breakthrough pain, a transient exacerbation of pain that occurs despite baseline analgesic therapy, requires prompt and effective intervention. Calculating rescue doses of analgesics is essential for providing rapid relief. Formulating a comprehensive pain management plan should include provisions for managing breakthrough pain.

Calculating dosages for pediatric and geriatric patients presents unique challenges. In pediatrics, weight-based dosing is common, and age-related considerations are paramount. In geriatric patients, age-related physiological changes, such as decreased renal and hepatic function, necessitate careful dosage adjustments. Polypharmacy, the concurrent use of multiple medications, is common in older adults and increases the risk of drug interactions. A comprehensive medication review is essential for optimizing pain management in this population. Pain assessment is an ongoing process that requires regular evaluation of the patient's pain level, functional status, and response to therapy. Utilizing validated pain scales, such as the numerical rating scale or the visual analog scale, can facilitate objective assessment. Effective communication between healthcare providers, patients, and caregivers is crucial for optimizing pain management.

www.ingramcontent.com/pod-product-compliance
Lightning Source LLC
LaVergne TN
LVHW022009200926
848481LV00007B/2296